OSTEONECROSIS

Edited by **Alessandro R Zorzi**
and **João Batista de Miranda**

Osteonecrosis
http://dx.doi.org/10.5772/63261
Edited by Alessandro R Zorzi and João Batista de Miranda

Contributors

Mario Pérez-Sayáns García, Carmen Vidal Real, José M Suárez Peñaranda, Abel García García, Kenji Yamagata, Ismet Gavrankapetanovic, Amel Hadzimehmedagic, Adnan Papovic, Mehmed Jamakosmanovic, Elizabeth Perez Hernandez, Eulalio Elizalde Martinez, Juan Manuel Torres Fernandez, Alessandro Rozim Zorzi

Published by InTech
Janeza Trdine 9, 51000 Rijeka, Croatia

Publishing Process Manager Iva Lipovic
Technical Editor SPi Global
Cover InTech Design team

First published June, 2017
Printed in Croatia
Legal deposit, Croatia: National and University Library in Zagreb

Additional hard copies can be obtained from orders@intechopen.com

Osteonecrosis, Edited by Alessandro R Zorzi and João Batista de Miranda
p. cm.
Print ISBN 978-953-51-3307-0
Online ISBN 978-953-51-3308-7

For EU product safety concerns:
IN TECH d.o.o., Prolaz Marije Krucifikse Kozulić 3, 51000 Rijeka, Croatia,
info@intechopen.com or visit our website at intechopen.com.

Meet the editors

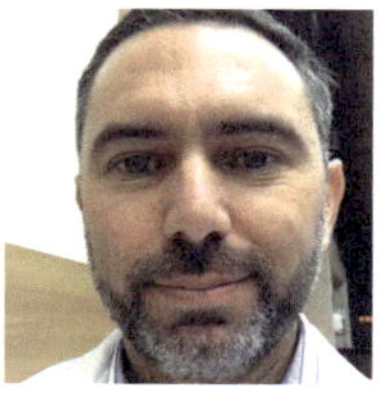

Dr. Alessandro R. Zorzi is an orthopedic surgeon at the University of Campinas (Unicamp, Brazil), where he practices surgeries, develops research, and teaches medical students, orthopedic fellows, and postgraduates. He obtained his MD degree at USP-Ribeirão Preto in 1999, his MSc degree at UNICAMP in 2010, a specialization in clinical research from Harvard Medical School in 2013, and his PhD degree at Unicamp in 2015. He is the author of dozens of international publications such as original articles, review articles, and book chapters. He is also the editor of the books *Bone Grafting* and *Advanced Techniques in Bone Regeneration*, both from InTech Open.

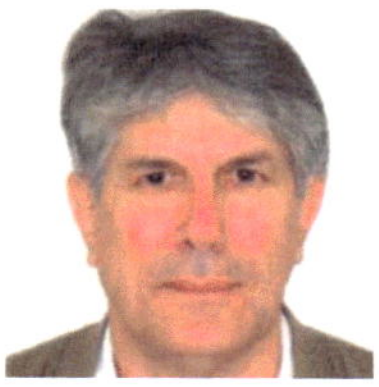

Professor João Batista de Miranda is the chairman of the Division of Knee Surgery and Inflammatory Diseases, at the Department of Orthopedic Surgery, Campinas State University (Unicamp), Brazil. He performs teaching activities with medical students, orthopedic fellows, and postgraduating researchers. He also develops research and clinical care. He is currently the superintendent of the Unicamp Teaching Hospital. Prof. Miranda obtained PhD with an experimental study on bone regeneration and on allografts. He has published several scientific articles in international journals and is coeditor of the book Bone Grafting of InTechOpen.

Contents

Preface

This book was born of another initiative of the publisher InTechOpen, one of the pioneers in the movement for free access to knowledge, called Open Access. Through its extensive network of contacts with researchers from several areas, the publisher invites authors to send chapters related to the chosen theme. After a thorough review, the best chapters are selected to compose the work, thus ensuring the quality of its content.

The etiology of osteonecrosis is still not fully understood, but one of the most respected theories is bone ischemia, leading to pain and deformity of the metaphyseal bone, causing joint deformity and incongruity. This often evolves into chronic pain and osteoarthritis. Many patients end up undergoing surgical treatments, such as knee and hip arthroplasties. However, other bones, such as the jaw and spinal vertebrae, received little attention in the past. The purpose of this book is to present updates on the treatment of osteonecrosis, and the reader will find in this book very interesting chapters on topics little discussed in the field of osteonecrosis.

Alessandro R Zorzi, MD, MSc, PhD
Department of Orthopedic Surgery
University of Campinas, Brazil

Section 1

Orthopedic Surgery and Rheumatology

Chapter 1

Introductory Chapter: Unusual Aspects of Osteonecrosis of the Human Skeleton

Alessandro Rozim Zorzi and
João Batista de Miranda

Additional information is available at the end of the chapter

http://dx.doi.org/10.5772/intechopen.69805

1. Introduction

Osteonecrosis, also called avascular necrosis or aseptic necrosis, is the name given to a set of diseases that affect mainly young adults and that often evolve to deformities and osteoarthritis, generating serious functional incapacity. The most affected site in the human skeleton is the head of the femur, but it can occur in many other places.

Despite advances in the understanding of this condition, the pathogenesis, risk factors, and diagnosis are not yet fully understood. In addition, the available treatments are still controversial and may range from physiotherapy and medications to surgical procedures such as decompression and arthroplasties [1].

Some authors report that osteonecrosis is responsible for at least 10% of the hip arthroplasties practiced in the United States [2].

2. Etiology

The term osteonecrosis means, "bone necrosis." Necrosis is a histopathological event that can occur after four types of injury:

1. Physical
2. Thermal
3. Toxic
4. Circulatory.

When we refer to osteonecrosis in orthopedics, we are actually using the term for circulatory lesions that affect the bone, which would be better called "infarction." Necrosis caused by circulatory injury may be due to

1. arterial diseases
2. embolism
3. venous obstruction.

In 1915, Phemister described and differentiated histological changes from necrosis caused by infection (septic necrosis) of those caused by circulatory changes (aseptic necrosis).

Regardless of the predisposing factor, the cause of osteonecrosis is always the inadequate blood perfusion of the bone [3]. Bone is a rigid and nondistensible tissue. Besides that, subchondral limited collateral circulation on the convex side of articular surfaces and decreased perfusion pressure of all epiphyses, which helps to explain the higher incidence of osteonecrosis in some regions of the skeleton.

3. Risk factors

Risk factors for osteonecrosis can be divided into three major groups, summarized in **Table 1**. When no risk factor is identified, osteonecrosis is called "primary."

Physical injury	Fractures Dislocations Surgeries Ionizing radiation Electric injuries Freezing
Lipid metabolism	Hypercortisolism Alcoholism Medication
Intraosseous hypertension	Dysbarism Gaucher's disease Sickle cell disease Autoimmune diseases

Table 1. Risk factors for "secondary" aseptic osteonecrosis [3].

4. Pathological anatomy

The following four stages of disease progression were identified [4]:

- Stage I: necrosis of bone and bone marrow without evidence of repair

- Stage II: repair at the periphery of the lesion
- Stage III: joint surface collapse
- Stage IV: secondary osteoarthritis.

5. Diagnosis

The diagnosis of osteonecrosis is made through clinical presentation and imaging tests.

The clinical history suggestive of osteonecrosis is the acute onset of severe pain in a patient who had no previous symptoms or who had mild chronic pain. Most of the time, there is no history of trauma associated with the onset of pain.

On physical examination, the affected area shows tenderness and edema. In deep joints, such as the shoulder and the hip, this can be difficult to observe. In addition, both active and passive movements of the affected joint are painful.

Among the imaging exams, the most commonly used are simple radiographies (X-ray), radionuclide scintigraphy (bone scan), and magnetic resonance imaging (MRI). Although bone scan can detect changes well before X-ray, these two methods can only detect reparative processes. Therefore, they can only diagnose from stage II of the disease. The advantage of MRI is that it can detect early bone marrow changes, still in stage I of the disease [3, 5].

6. Clinical presentations

6.1. Hip

Femoral head osteonecrosis is the most common site affected by osteonecrosis and perhaps the best studied. About 20% of the cases are idiopathic. The rest are linked to alcoholism, corticosteroid therapy, and other factors already described in **Table 1**. Surgical treatment varies. In mild or moderate cases, there is the possibility of preserving the joint with techniques such as decompression, osteotomies, bone grafting, and new stem cell therapies. Severe cases should be treated with arthroplasties, which can vary in partial or total arthroplasties and resurfacing [6].

An important aspect related to osteonecrosis of the hip is the vascularization of the head of the femur and the changes that this vascularization presents throughout life. In this sense, Ismet Gavrankapetanović and co-authors present us, in this book, a very interesting chapter on this topic, addressing an unexplored topic, which is the relationship between hip development disorder and osteonecrosis.

6.2. Knee

In addition to the traditional osteonecrosis itself, two other entities must be recognized: spontaneous osteonecrosis of the knee (SPONK) described by Ahlback in 1968 and postoperative osteonecrosis (ONPK) described by Brahme in 1991.

Patients with SPONK have a different epidemiological profile, since they affect women over 50 in only one joint, with a single small lesion, without the traditional risk factors (use of corticosteroids, alcoholism, etc.).

Similarly, ONPK has an epidemiological profile similar to SPONK, only occurring after a surgical intervention, which is most often an arthroscopic meniscectomy indicated for meniscal degenerative lesions. Anterior Cruciate Ligament (ACL) surgery and cartilage procedures also could predispose to ONPK.

The current trend is to consider SPONK and ONPK as subchondral bone insufficiency fractures, unlike osteonecrosis, which is caused by a bone infarct [7].

6.3. Ankle

The site most affected by osteonecrosis in the foot and ankle segment is the talus. The most frequent etiology is trauma (75%). Osteonecrosis is a complication well known and feared in the treatment of talus fractures because of the precarious vascular supply of this bone.

One of the ways to treat and prevent osteonecrosis of the talus is through early and accurate anatomic reduction. Once osteonecrosis is established, the first measure is limited weight bearing. In the failure of this treatment, the surgery is indicated, being basically divided into two groups: the arthrodesis and the ankle arthroplasty [8].

6.4. Shoulder

Osteonecrosis of the humeral head (ONHH) is an uncommon condition, but after the hip, it is the second most common site of nontraumatic osteonecrosis. The four-part fracture is the most common cause of ONHH.

The most widely used classification is the Cruess classification system, which has five stages according to radiographic appearance as follows:

Stage I: normal X-ray with altered MRI;

Stage II: sclerotic bone without collapse;

Stage III: crescent sign;

Stage IV: collapse of the humeral head;

Stage V: osteoarthritis.

Treatment could be divided as nonoperative, arthroscopic debridement, core decompression, bone grafting, and shoulder arthroplasty [9].

6.5. Elbow

The elbow is rarely affected by osteonecrosis. According to Le et al. [10], the most affected sites are the capitellum and the lateral epicondyles, being, therefore, a rare differential diagnosis of tennis elbow syndrome.

6.6. Wrist

Osteonecrosis of the wrist most commonly involves the scaphoid, lunate, and capitate. Scaphoid is the most frequently injured bone in the carpus. It is second only to the femoral head in the incidence of posttraumatic osteonecrosis. In the absence of trauma, it is known as Preiser's disease [11].

Osteonecrosis of the lunate is known as Kienbock's disease. It is associated with trauma, overuse, and negative ulnar variance [11].

Osteonecrosis of the capitate is a rare condition and often associated with trauma.

6.7. Spine

Osteonecrosis of the vertebral body is also known as Kummel's disease (KD), usually related to osteoporotic vertebral fractures. It is a rare and under diagnosed disease. Elizabeth Pérez Hernández and co-authors gave us a rare chapter on this subject in this book.

6.8. Jaw

Unlike orthopedics, where the term osteonecrosis has been used for pathologies resulting from aseptic bone infarction, in dentistry, the term is used in its broadest sense, indicating the death of the bony tissue. Recently, the problem of osteonecrosis caused by the use of medicines, known by the abbreviation MRONJ, has gained much interest.

In this book, Kenji Yamagata and Mario Pérez-Sayáns García present chapters that address in depth of this relevant and current topic.

6.9. Multifocal osteonecrosis

When three or more separate articulations are involved, concurrently or consecutively, it is called a multifocal osteonecrosis (MFON).

The most common cause of MFON is the use of corticosteroids [5]. It is therefore important to have a high degree of suspicion in patients on chronic use of this medication that present more than one site of involvement in X-ray. Bone scintigraphy may be helpful in these cases, as some sites, such as the shoulders, may be little symptomatic at the beginning, when preservation strategies of the joint, such as decompression, have its indication.

7. Conclusion

Publications regarding osteonecrosis rarely provide an overview of the problem. In general, the subject is included as a chapter on books that address some specific joints, such as osteonecrosis of the hip and osteonecrosis of the knee.

Works dedicated to dealing with the subject also usually give greater prominence to the novelties related to the articulations of greater prevalence.

Although succinct, the aim of this book is to highlight some recent or little discussed topics of the subject, hardly present in other works. In this sense, the reader will find very interesting chapters, written by several specialists who deal in research and clinical practice with the set of problems called osteonecrosis.

Author details

Alessandro Rozim Zorzi* and João Batista de Miranda

*Address all correspondence to: alessandrozorzi@uol.com.br

Department of Orthopedic Surgery, State University of Campinas, Campinas, Brazil

References

[1] Marker DR, Mont MA, Seyler TM, LaPorte DM, Frassica FJ. Current literature: An educational tool to study osteonecrosis for the orthopaedic in-training examination?. Orthopedic Clinics of North America. 2009;**40**:299-304

[2] Jackson SM, Major NM. Pathologic conditions mimicking osteonecrosis. Orthopedic Clinics of North America. 2004;**35**:315-320

[3] Bullough PG, DiCarlo EF. Subchondral avascular necrosis: A common cause of arthritis. Annals of the Rheumatic Diseases. 1990;**49**:412-420

[4] Ficat RP, Arlet J. Ischemia and Necrosis of Bone. Baltimore: Williams and Wilkins; 1980

[5] Sun W, Shi Z, Gao F, Wang B, Li Z. The pathogenesis of multifocal osteonecrosis. Scientific Reports. 2016;**6**:29576

[6] Babis GC, Soucacos PN. Effectiveness of total hip arthroplasty in the management of hip osteonecrosis. Orthopedic Clinics of North America. 2004;**35**:359-364

[7] Yamamoto T, Bullough PJ. Spontaneous osteonecrosis of the knee: the result of subchondral insufficiency fracture. Journal of Bone and Joint Surgery American Volume. 2000; **82**:858-866

[8] Adelaar RS, Madrian JR. Avascular necrosis of the talus. Orthopedic Clinics of North America. 2004;**35**:383-395

[9] Sarris J, Weiser R, Sotereanos DG. Pathogenesis and treatment of osteonecrosis of the shoulder. Orthopedic Clinics of North America. 2004;**35**:397-404

[10] Le TB, Mont MA, Jones LC, LaPorte DM, Hungerford DS. Atraumatic osteonecrosis of the adult elbow. Clinical Orthopaedics and Related Research. 2000;**373**:141-145

[11] Botte MJ, Pacelli LL, Gelberman RH. Vascularity and osteonecrosis of the wrist. Orthopedic Clinics of North America. 2004;**35**:405-421

Chapter 2

Osteonecrosis and Hip Development Disorder

Ismet Gavrankapetanović, Amel Hadžimehmedagić,
Adnan Papović and Mehmed Jamakosmanović

Additional information is available at the end of the chapter

http://dx.doi.org/10.5772/intechopen.68161

Abstract

Blood vessel branching of the proximal femur by its scheme differs from all other major joints. This scheme changes during the individual's development, dynamically depending on age. Namely, the caliber, blood flow rate, and dominance of certain arteries from the entire network of blood vessels that participate in the vascular supply of the hip are not equally expressed in all stages of development. In each successive stage, blood supply is dominated by a different artery that, after a certain period of time, shifts its major role to another artery. Anastomoses between individual arteries are not constant in all stages of development, and they represent a great importance for compensatory mechanisms. The disturbance of local arterial blood vessels, at a time when they dominate the blood supply and affect the quality of hip development and maturation, leads to reduced perfusion, and consequently, to the lack of development, ossification, and possible osteonecrosis.

Keywords: osteonecrosis, hip developmental disorder, bone, hip vascular supply

1. Introduction

Blood vessel branching of the proximal femur by its scheme differs from all other major joints. This scheme changes during the individual's development, dynamically depending on age. Namely, the caliber, blood flow rate, and dominance of certain arteries from the entire network of blood vessels that participate in hip vascular supply are not equally expressed in all stages of development. In each successive stage, blood supply is dominated by a different artery that, after a certain period of time, shifts its major role to another artery. Anastomoses between individual arteries are not constant in all stages of development, and they represent a great importance for compensatory mechanisms. The disturbance of local arterial blood vessels, at a time when they dominate the blood supply and affect the quality of hip development and maturation, leads to reduced perfusion, and consequently, to the lack of development, ossification, and possible osteonecrosis.

The problem of the circulation and vascular network supplying bones is exposed as a main problem in the etiology and pathogenesis of hip disorders in children which can affect later stages of life. The authentication of the problem is quite hard since bone biology is inappropriate for the assessment of vascular status. Results and first signs of diseases are visible after a couple of months or even longer.

Acute or chronic ischemia in other tissues has a specific clinical presentation and symptomatology, which is not the case with the hip joint. Also, techniques that are applicable for vascular status assessment in other tissues are almost useless for the estimation of the vascular status on bone tissue.

2. Bone vascular system

As in other tissues, vascular system of the bones can be divided into three levels: afferent and efferent blood vessel and a microvascular network that fills in the space between them (**Figure 1**). Afferent blood vessel is composed of epiphyseal, metaphyseal, nutrient, and periosteal arteries. Microvascular network consists of medullar sinusoid, cortical, and periosteal capillaries, while the efferent blood vessel is formed of epiphyseal, metaphyseal, nutrient and periosteal veins, and collective sinusoids. None of the mentioned vascular elements can be considered independent. There are numerous anastomoses between them and opinions about one's participation in bone nutrition are still divided.

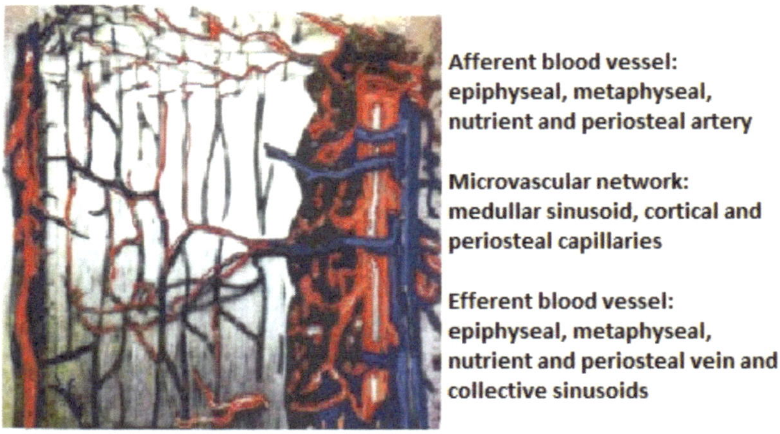

Figure 1. Bone vascularization.

http://dx.doi.org/10.5772/intechopen.68161

The nutrient artery is the main artery supplying the cortex of the bone. Its branches separate under a sharp angle and do not divide further. In medullar cavity, the nutrient artery is divided into ascendant and descendant medullar arteries. Branches separate radially out of these supply cortices. In normal bone structure, there is a centrifugal flow meaning that blood vessel interchange is parallel to Haver's channels and bone axis. These blood vessels drain into venules on the periosteal bone surface. This type of vascular organization has functional meaning allowing relatively high intramedullary pressure that can affect movements of the interstitial fluid in bones [1].

3. Specificity of hip vascular supply

Blood supply of the hip is specific. It is formed of rich vascular network, that is, in great deal, responsible for the development of the joint. Blood vessels that participate in the hip vascularization can be divided into nutritive, retinacular, and foveolar. Retinacular blood vessels are the main source of hip supply and are extremely vulnerable (**Figures 2** and **3**). They can be damaged by infection, joint fluid, trauma, or forced position of the joint. Blood supply of the hip changes and adjusts during joint stages of development, from embryonal to the adolescent stage, when it adopts definite appearance and functional characteristics. Stages of vascular supply of the hip consist of fetal, infantile, intermediary, prepuberty, adolescent, and adult stage [2]. Each stage is different by the role of main nutritive artery of the diaphysis, metaphysis, periosteal, and anastomoses. The only constant factor in all of the mentioned stages is that the supplying blood vessels come from the a. femoralis communis, a. profundae femoris, and branched of the a. iliacae internae—a. gluteae and a. obturatoriae. The most important artery for hip supply is a. profunda femoris with its branches—a. circumflexa femoris medialis and lateralis.

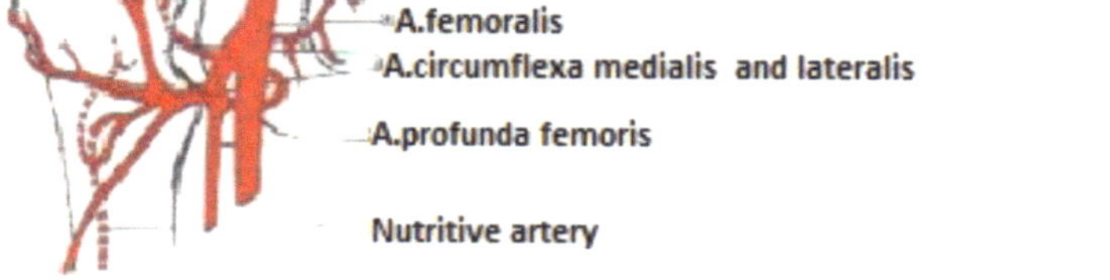

Figure 2. Scheme of arteries of the coxofemoral region.

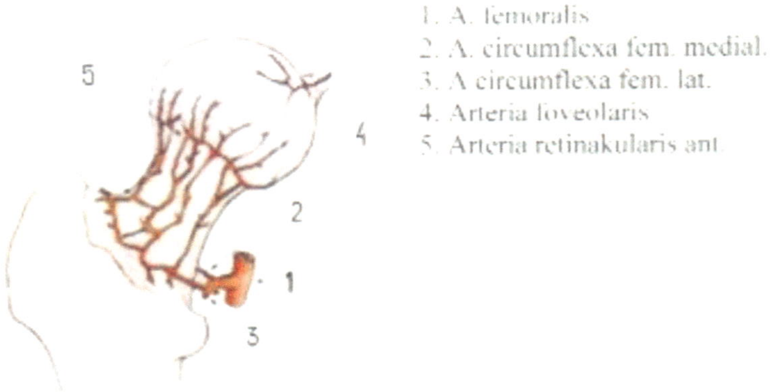

Figure 3. Scheme of arterial blood supply of the femoral head and neck (anterior view).

Final branches of the a. circumflexae femoris medialis and lateralis form anastomoses that together with a. obturatoria and a. glutealis make circulus arteriosus—arterial ring around the femoral neck (**Figure 4**). This ring can be found pericapsullary as well as intracapsullary. From extracapsular arterial ring, retinacular arteries are formed that diverge in regular interval and pass through capsule forming ascendant cervical arteries. These arteries, by their position, can be divided into anterior, posterior, medial, and lateral, and their function is to supply femoral head and neck. Extracapsular ring forms medial metaphyseal and lateral epiphyseal arteries that supply blood to epiphyseal gap. These nutritional arteries pass through the capsule in the lower lateral part of the femoral neck parallel with intertrochanteric line where arterial circulation can be jeopardized leading to avascular necrosis (AVN) of the femoral head.

The intracapsular arterial ring is positioned subsynovially around the distal part of the femoral neck. This ring forms vascular borderline of the joint (circulus articuli vasculorum

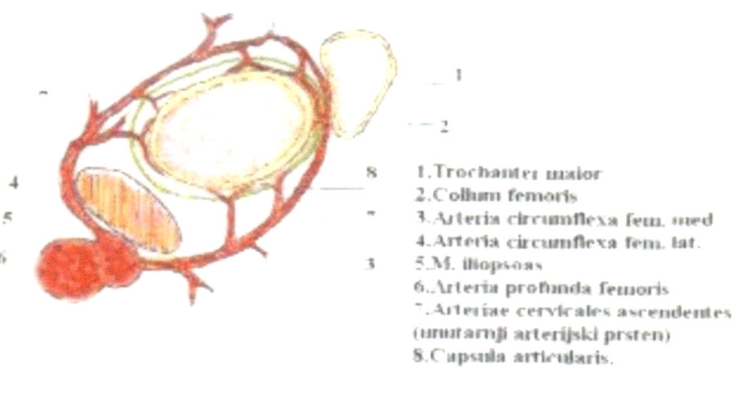

Figure 4. Scheme of extracapsular and intracapsular arterial ring.

Hunteri). Out of this ring, short arteries depart to the bone metaphysis or articular cartilage of the femoral head in which ossification nuclei end. Every artery supplies only one ossification nucleus. In the case where there are multiple secondary ossification nuclei, every one of them is supplied by separate artery that anastomoses in between which can explain partial necrosis of the femoral head [3].

4. Dynamics of development of hip blood supply

Dynamics of hip development blood supply are intensified by movements in the joint through stages of development of a person. The entire dynamic process can be divided into five phases:

(a) *Fetal phase* includes the entire intrauterine period and first 4 months of life. A. circumflexa femoris medialis and lateralis together with a. obturatoria give outer epiphyseal, ascendant, and lower metaphyseal arteries. In this stage morphologically and functionally a. circumflexa femoris lateralis is more developed. Outer epiphyseal arteries are directed horizontally and by the inner part of the femoral head. Lower and ascendant metaphyseal arteries have vertical flow. Their branches are directed toward the inner side of one part of the femoral head, while foveolar arteries pass through ligament capitis femoris supplying the inner part of the femoral head.

(b) *Infantile phase* is considered from 4 months of life to 4 years of age. The most intensive growth and development of the collateral blood vessels that form arterial ring around the femoral neck occur between the sixth and the 18th month of life. This stage coincides with the walking phase that is considered the most intensive period for the establishment of physiological motions in the hip joint. In this phase, epiphyseal arteries get stronger, getting their supply from a. circumflexa femoris medialis that takes over the dominant role for blood supply. There are no arteries that pass through ligament capitis femoris, and anastomoses that amplify supply through arterial ring around the femoral neck are poorly developed.

(c) *Intermediary phase* is considered from 4 to 7 years of age. In this phase, epiphyseal vessels are constant with significant caliber, while metaphyseal vessels fall behind in development. The characteristic of this phase is the strengthening of the arteries of ligament capitis femoris. This phase includes the development of the arterial ring around the femoral neck.

(d) *Prepuberty phase* includes period between the eighth and the 10th years of life where definite development is dominating with stabilization of all, already, formed anastomoses.

(e) *Adolescent phase* is considered on a period between the 11th and the 15th years of life when, regarding vascular system, metaphyseal blood vessel network is established and when growth of the proximal femur is ended. In this stage, outer epiphyseal arteries and a. capitis femoris are leading the blood supply and are basis for arterial network of the femoral head and neck in adults [4–6].

5. Avascular necrosis as a consequence of treatment of developmental hip dysplasia (DDH)

5.1. AVN: complication or inevitable consequence of the treatment of DDH?

AVN in different degrees is a well-known complication of the treatment of DDH. It can be a devastating complication with possible premature development of osteoarthrosis. In a milder degree, it can be manifested through minimal residual deformity and hip dysfunction.

5.2. Definition of AVN

It is quite hard to define AVN. Weinstein, instead of the term AVN, used a term "growth disorder of the proximal femur" [7]. However, when milder degrees of AVN are analyzed, this term is not suitable because there is no actual growth disorder. This is the most serious complication connected with the treatment of hip development disorder. Its sequelae are deformity of the femoral head, permanent acetabular dysplasia with chronic lateral subluxation, relative hypotrophy of the great trochanter, and abbreviation of the lower extremities.

In fact, AVN represents complication of bone blood supply in terms of inadequate perfusion and oxygenation; it is extremely rare in healthy children, while it is quite often in children with diagnosed hip development disorder. AVN is characterized, on a microscopic level, by zones of devitalized bone trabecula and bone marrow that have tendency to spread and affect the subchondral plate. From the entire proximal femur, its head is the most vulnerable spot for the development of AVN. The most common position of the development of AVN is just below the joint cartilage that was affected by ischemia the most or suffers the greatest pressure which is the anterolateral aspect of the femoral head. However, there is no specific part of the femoral head that is spared of the affect of AVN. In adult patients, where in childhood had diagnosed hip development disorder and noted AVN, the affected segment was never totally revascularized. Once detected, collapse of the femoral head usually persists [8–10].

The beginning of disease is inconvincible and practically asymptomatic. AVN usually progresses until complete destruction of the joint that, even before the fifth decade of life, demands radical surgery—hip joint replacement. It is estimated that 10% of 500,000 hip replacement surgeries performed in the USA per year have indication of AVN.

5.3. Pathophysiology of the AVN in DDH

Pathological changes that can lead to the development of the AVN have their beginning in two different categories: vascular and extra vascular factors. Vascular factors can be divided into arterial and vein factors.

5.3.1. Vascular factors

All vascular factors can be divided into arterial and vein factors. Almost all vascular factors are located extraosseally. Arterial factors are, probably, the dominant and most important

http://dx.doi.org/10.5772/intechopen.68161

factors for the development of the AVN. The femoral head is, because of the arteries that are marked as arteries of the terminal type and their relatively bad developed collateral network, a part of the body that is most liable to development of the AVN. Some kind of trauma that hip suffers during the surgery, in order to achieve optimal relations in coxofemoral joint, can lead toward thrombosis with contusion or even complete interruption of lateral retinacular arteries that in the critical period are basic for blood supply of the femoral head and neck. Compared to other tissues, such incident can be marked as only infarction that covers the irrigational spot of the affected blood vessel. In children with hip development disorder, a less valuable hip is noted and in most cases with weaker developed blood vessels. During treatment of this kind of a hip, possible attenuation of vascular network can be seen. In older patients that have been diagnosed with DDH, atherosclerotic changes can be presented on magisterial as well as on terminal arteries of this region. In middle-aged female patients, vasculitis and Raynaud's disease can lead toward exacerbation of the AVN, while in male patients, AVN is expressed after decompression or because of vasospasm.

Those rare vascular factors that act intraosseously are related to vein blood flow and are less often caused by intraosseal arterial events. Primer etiological factor for the development of the AVN in this group is micro-embolism. Micro-embolism in one irrigational field blocks circulation in one part of the femoral head. This condition can be seen in cases of fat embolism, air embolism, or thrombosis, while steroid therapy is administered. Intraosseal vascular factors refer to all diseases that reduce vein blood outflow causing vein stasis. All types of vein stasis, because of increase of pressure, can indirectly lead to AVN. Some metabolic or hormonal disruption leads to the enlargement of intramedullary fat-loading osteocytes. This directly influences shift in space and reduction of vein capacity resulting in difficulties with vein drainage. Intraosseal phlebography that was performed in patients with AVN showed abnormalities in drainage system emphasizing the fact that vein circulation participated in development and contributed in the progression of this disease. Capability of decompression in space occupied with bone marrow depends on regional anatomical structures especially of vascular outflow and bone architecture. The femoral head, unfortunately, does not have anatomical advantages as other bones because of its formation as a socket on a narrow metaphyseal neck. Only a couple of vein channels go through bone cortex and have the capability of direct decompression. Increased pressure during disproportion in inflow and outflow has to be directed toward narrow metaphyseal neck [11–14].

5.3.2. Extravascular factors

Intraosseal factors are basic factors that influence the development of AVN from this group. Skeletal system in subchondral zone of the femoral head is a closed rigid cortical socket. This system is conditionally sensitive on pressure increase that can result in somewhat like a compartment syndrome. Many authors have described the increase of the pressure in bone marrow of the proximal femur in many patients diagnosed with AVN. First effects of pressure increase can be resulted in vein outflow, sinusoids, and small capillaries. Reflex spasm can even block nutritive arteries before they reach cortex. The subchondral zone of the femoral head that is in most intimate contact with acetabulum is not in a favorable position because of the mechanical relations. Pressure and friction on one side together with weaker blood supply create a baffle effect that can contribute to further restriction of the decompression of bone marrow in the affected region opposite of subchondral zones with regular perfusion. Trabecular deformity, which can occur because of this kind of development also compresses medullar space and leads to an increase in the intraosseal pressure. This kind of situation can contribute to morphological changes, reduction of trabecula, thinning of bone matrix, and disturbance in dynamics of ossification. An increase of the bone pressure strives to concentrate in the affected zone because of specificity of its architecture. This process, together with an increase of the intraosseal pressure, tends to transform ischemic zone that was marginally affected into the zone of complete bone infarction with functional anoxia [15].

5.4. Pathophysiology of the AVN

Macroscopic changes of the AVN on the femoral head show a thin layer of compact subchondral bone and joint cartilage. Joint cartilage can be supplied with synovial fluid. The only part of cartilage that can lead to necrosis is around the zone of demarcation. Bone part of the femoral head can lead to necrosis in the form of irregular areas of yellowish necrosis, while only some of trabeculae seem vital. In progression of the process, spot-like zones of necrosis start to resorb which can be seen on X-rays. In further development, micro-fractures can be noticed and consequently bone sequesters start to form. The line of the trabecular fracture goes through necrotic part of the bone-causing formation of joint sequester. Because of this, the affected region of the femoral head collapses. After this, progressive destruction of joint cartilage is noted with formation of free joint bodies (corpora libera) and marginal osteophytes.

From pathophysiological aspect, AVN can be divided into phase of cellular necrosis and phase of reparation.

Cellular necrosis first affects hematopoietic elements (6–12 h after insult), after which necrosis of bone cells follows: osteocytes, osteoblasts, and osteoclasts (12–48 h after insult), followed by necrosis of fat cells of bone marrow (2–5 days after insult). Complete absence of osteocytes in localized areas of trabecular bone is real indicator of the existence of AVN. This is a typical finding for AVN that lasts 14 days. Phase of death of fat cells of bone marrow can be recognized by vacuoles inside a cell that do not have a nucleus, thus looking alike to lipoid cysts. Bone infarction can be recognized into four zones: central zone of cellular necrosis surrounded by concentrically circles of ischemia, hyperemia, and zone of normal tissue. Once AVN is noticed, products of necrotic tissue cause initial inflammatory response that is manifested with vasodilatation, fluid transudation, fibrin precipitation, and local leukocytes infiltration. This response is the basis for the development of hyperemia and the basis for the start of reparatory process—reconstruction of infarct zone. In reparatory phase, bone resorption is noted first that is followed by a neoosification process. The reparatory phase does not happen inside of the necrotic and ischemic zone, but between vital and infracted zone, because it demands adequate perfusion. Reparatory response results in progressive growth of reactive border that demarks that part of the bone tissue that is doomed to failure. Mesenchyme cells and capillary proliferation supply macrophages and fibroblasts entrance into "dead zone," which starts the reparatory phase that is presented as osteoporosis. Progressive loss of mechanical support and destruction of bone architecture are trying to be replaced by the activity of osteoblasts which is usually not enough because this process is followed by micro-fractures on places with least resistance. Fractures, fragmentations, and other disorders on the subchondral bone are visible signs of this process on normal X-ray. Capillary invasion extends to the subchondral part of the bone tissue and resorbs cartilage. This phase used to hold conviction in many orthopedic surgeons for osteochondritis dissecans [16–19].

5.5. Consequences of the AVN

Consequences of AVN can be divided into minimal and manifest changes [19]. If irrigational zone of occluded blood vessel is small and does not cover large amount of space with supply, patients can have minimal changes with insignificant or even no symptoms at all. These changes get detected rarely or accidentally through some diagnostic procedure for some other disease. Because of this, many patients do not get included into studies about AVN and its consequences. On the other side, manifest changes become visible when multiple occlusions on blood vessels are formed. These changes on specific bone regions become visible on X-rays after certain period of time. Signs of bone change are noticeable in the form of necrosis that subjects to slow but limited reparatory process. In the background, reactive zone of reparation is visible that forms sclerotic edge of trabecular thickening. These reparatory attempts can be followed and noticeable through different stages as well as different forms of necrosis and remodeling.

Author details

Ismet Gavrankapetanović[1]*, Amel Hadžimehmedagić[2], Adnan Papović[1] and Mehmed Jamakosmanović[1]

*Address all correspondence to: ismetcap@ortotrauma.com.ba

1 Clinic for Orthopedics and Traumatology, University Clinical Center Sarajevo, Sarajevo, Bosnia and Herzegovina

2 Clinic for Vascular Surgery, University Clinical Center Sarajevo, Sarajevo, Bosnia and Herzegovina

References

[1] Stewart K, Edmonds-Wilson R, Brand R, Brown T. Spatial distribution of hip capsule structural and material properties. Journal of Biomechanics. 2002;**35**(11):1491-1498

[2] Trueta J. The normal vascular anatomy of the normal human femoral head during growth. The Journal of Bone and Joint Surgery. 1957;**39**(2):358-394

[3] Schunke M, et al. Nutrition of the femoral head. Atlas of Anatomy. Thieme. 2006;382-389

[4] Ogden JA. Changing patterns of proximal femoral vascularity. JBJS. 1974;**56**:941-950

[5] Damsin JP, Lazennec JY, Gonzales M, Guerin-Surville H, Hannoun L. Arterial supply of the acetabulum in the fetus: Application to periacetabular surgery in childhood. Surgical and Radiologic Anatomy. 1992;**14**(3):215-221

[6] Chung SM. The arterial supply of the developing proximal end of the human femur. The Journal of Bone and Joint Surgery. 1976;**58**(7):961-970

[7] Weinstein SL. Developmental hip dysplasia. Lovell and Winter's Pediatric Orthopaedics. 1996

[8] Ilfeld FW, O'Hara J, Robins G, et al. Congenital dislocation of the hip. Clinical Orthopaedics. 1972;**86**:21-27

[9] Gage JR, Winter RB. Avascular necrosis of the capital femoral epiphysis as complication of closed reduction of congenital dislocation of the hip. A critical review of twenty years experience at Gillette Children's Hospital. Journal of Bone and Joint Surgery. 1972;**54**(A):373-388

[10] Cooperman DR, Wallensten R, Stulberg SD. Post-reduction avascular necrosis in congenital dislocation of the hip. Journal of Bone and Joint Surgery. 1980;**62**(A):247-258

[11] Glueck CJ, Freiberg RA, Wang P. Role of thrombosis in osteonecrosis. Current Hematology Reports. 2003;**2**(5):417-422

[12] Mont MA, Hungerford DS. Non-traumatic avascular necrosis of the femoral head. Journal of Bone and Joint Surgery American Volume. 1995;**77**:459-474

[13] Heringou P, Habibi A, Bachir D, Galacteros F. The natural history of asymptomatic osteonecrosis of the femoral head in adults with sickle cell disease. Journal of Bone and Joint Surgery American Volume. 2006;**88**(12):2565-2572

[14] Drescher W, Li H, Lundgaard A, Bunger C, Hansen ES. Endothelin-1-induced femoral head epiphyseal artery constriction is enhanced by long-term corticosteroid treatment. Journal of Bone and Joint Surgery American Volume. 2006;**88**(3):173-179

[15] Watson R, Roach N, Dalinka M. Avascular necrosis and bone marrow edema syndrome. Radiologic Clinics of North America. **42**(1):207-219

[16] Aaron RK, Dyke JP, Ciombor DM, Ballon D, Lee J, Jung E, Tung GA. Perfusion abnormalities in subchondral bone associated with marrow edema, osteoarthritis and avascular necrosis. Annals of the New York Academy of Sciences. 2007;**11**(17):124-137

[17] Connolly P, Weinstein SL. The course and treatment of avascular necrosis of the femoral head in developmental dysplasia of the hip. Acta Orthopaedica et Traumatologica Turcica. 2007;**41**(1):54-59

[18] Kerachian MA, Harvey EJ, Cournoyer D, Chow TY, Seguin C. Avascular necrosis of the femoral head: Vascular hypotheses. Endothelium. 2006;**13**(4):237-244

[19] Lafforgue P. Pathophysiology and natural history of avascular necrosis of bone. Joint Bone Spine. 2006;**73**(5):500-507

Chapter 3

Vertebral Osteonecrosis

Elizabeth Pérez Hernández,
Eulalio Elizalde Martínez and
Juan Manuel Torres Fernández

Additional information is available at the end of the chapter

http://dx.doi.org/10.5772/intechopen.69275

Abstract

Vertebral osteonecrosis (ON) is a rare, underdiagnosed disease, also called pseudarthrosis due to ischemia following a compression fracture (CF). The main features include the air-occupied intravertebral cleft visualized as a radiolucent shade of linear or semilunar X-ray, namely an intravertebral vacuum cleft (IVC) sign. Usually, this phenomenon shows low signal intensity with all magnetic resonance imaging (MRI) sequences. Another feature of ON of the vertebral body is the intravertebral fluid analogous to edema and fibrosis in histological sections. This appears as low signal intensity on T1-weighted MRI, with high signal intensity on T2-weighted images. The risk factors for vertebral ON are multivariate, and the pathophysiological mechanisms are still unknown with certainty.

Keywords: osteonecrosis, avascular necrosis, pseudarthrosis, Kümmel's disease, ischemia

1. Introduction

Necrosis of bone tissue is a nonspecific term that is related to conditions that cause major cell stress and cell death regularly due to interruption of the vascular supply. Frequently osteonecrosis (ON) is related to local traumatic events such as fractures that induce vascular injury; however, several non-traumatic causes have also been related. The first publications of ON were referred to avascular necrosis (AVN) of the femoral head and related in most cases to trauma. Later, other etiological factors were involved in the development of ON such as alcohol consumption, fat embolism, and steroid therapy. Likewise, coagulopathies, chronic osteoarthropathies, bone infections, and tumors are also causal factors associated with it.

AVN, aseptic necrosis, ischemic necrosis, subchondral AVN, and osteochondritis dissecans are synonyms used to denote ON. Vertebral AVN has been classically related to the intravertebral vacuum cleft (IVC) sign. This is represented by a transversal cleft of the vertebral body occupied by gas density observed in extension and not observed in flexion. Subsequently, with the advent of magnetic resonance imaging (MRI), the presence of fluid was demonstrated in association with osteoporotic vertebral collapse. In addition, ischemia was confirmed by histological analysis.

AVN of bone is otherwise characterized by massive necrosis of bone and bone marrow. This has been generally related to systemic factors such as alcohol abuse, glucocorticoid therapy, dyslipidemia, Gaucher disease or human immunodeficiency virus (HIV) infection, among others. AVN of the spine is known as Kümmel's disease (KD), usually related to osteoporotic vertebral fractures. Although the AVN associated with vertebral collapse hypothetically is a consequence of vascular damage, the pathogenesis, as well as the early diagnosis, the management protocols and prevention measures continue to be the research topics.

2. Historical background

AVN frequently associated with vertebral compression fractures (CF) in osteoporosis is called KD, first described by Herman Kümmell, a German surgeon in 1895. Also at that time, A.A. Verneuil, French, referred to some clinical cases with similar manifestations, so that occasionally this syndrome was named "Kümmell-Verneuil disease." The cases described by Kümmel had a history of minor spinal trauma, with asymptomatic periods from months to years and angular kyphotic spinal deformities of the lower thoracic or upper lumbar regions and the T12 segment with progressive painful [1, 2]. Kümmell hypothesized that there was no traumatic CF in all the patients; however, it seemed very likely that most of them had a history of minimal trauma with influence on local nutrition and progressive atrophy [3]. It should be mentioned that these observations described by Kümmell were performed before the advent of X-rays, and once these were used, the existence of the disease was questioned in "normal" radiographic studies with uncertain quality. Years later, the collapse of the delayed vertebral body was demonstrated; however, diagnostic criteria in the early stages of the disease were associated with negative radiographic findings [2, 4, 5].

Steel also classified the KD in five progressive stages [2]. Initially, it is characterized by hyperflexion of the radiographically normal vertebral column, namely, the *initial insult*. Subsequently, a second *post-traumatic stage* is categorized by minimal manifestations of the low back without functional limitation. This is followed by a *latent stage*, relative well-being, lasting weeks to months, with no significant symptoms. Then, the *stage of recrudescence*, the patient manifests pain in the back, develops gibbous and loss of progressive stature, in addition to peripheral pain. In the *terminal stage*, the patient develops a progressive back pain located in the region of the pathological fracture with angular kyphosis and compression of the spinal [2]. The cases of AVN without a history of spinal trauma should not be termed KD. **Table 1** summarizes the clinical cases of KD reported in the literature.

A frequently representative feature of vertebral ON has been named IVC sign. This was first described as a horizontal cleft with gas density in radiographic studies [6]. This entity has

http://dx.doi.org/10.5772/intechopen.69275

Age (years)	Sex	Location	Concomitant pathologies	Management	Reference
23/28/62	Male	T10/L1/T8	None	Immobilized in hyperextension	Steel [2]
71	Male	T12	Osteopenia Occasional alcohol abuse	Unknown	Brower and Downey [14]
45	Female	L1	Type 1 Gaucher disease	Conservative	Hermann et al. [15]
75	Male	T11	Steroids	Conservative	Van Eenenaam and el-Khoury [11]
72	Male	L4	Diabetes mellitus type II	Subtotal corpectomy/autologous grafting/ posterior fusion with pedicle fixation	Young et al. [7]
79	Male	L2	Chronic steroid therapy /myasthenia gravis	Conservative	Osterhouse and Kettner [16]
71	Female	L3	None	Posterior stabilization	Kapoor et al. [17]
62	Female	L2, L3	Osteopenia, diabetes	Unknown	Maheshwari et al. [18]
55	Male	L2	Sarcoidosis	Anterior decompression/L-2 corpectomy/ anterior L1–3 spinal fusion/autologous grafting	Ito et al. [19]
60	Male	T9-T10	Diabetes mellitus type II, chronic obstructive pulmonary disease, obesity, hypothyroidism secondary to radiation treatment for Graves' disease, and depression	T9 and T10 corpectomies with T8–T11 anterior and posterior fusion/cage graft with pedicle screw fixation	Swartz and Fee [20]
87	Female	L1	None	L1 vertebroplasty	Van der Schaaf and Fransen [21]
75	Female	T12	Dementia, Diabetes mellitus type 2, hypertension, hypothyroidism	T12 vertebroplasty	Ma et al. [5]
31	Male	L1	None	L1 kyphoplasty	Matzaroglou et al. [22]
81	Female	L1	Osteoporosis, obesity, idiopathic pulmonary thromboembolic, arterial hypertension, depression	Conservative (teriparatide)	Fabbriciani et al. [23]
60	Male	L4	Osteopenia	L4 laminectomy, L3-5/transpedicular fixation	Ranjan et al. [24]

Table 1. Case reports of Kümmel's disease since 1951.

also been called post-traumatic vertebral ON [3, 5, 7], IVC [8, 9], vertebral pseudarthrosis [10], delayed post-traumatic vertebral body collapse [11, 12] and nonunion of VCF [10, 13].

3. Clinical manifestations

KD occurs more frequently in the middle and in the elderly slightly predominant in males [7]. The incidence of KD in elderly patients ranges from 7 to 37%. One of the characteristic symptoms is an acute pain especially in the early stages of the disease usually without accompanying neurological symptomatology. In these cases, falls are generally conditioning factors of pain. The kyphotic deformity associated with recurrent pain of greater intensity in later stages usually corresponds to the collapse of the vertebral bodies and is usually located in the thoracolumbar region. Then neurological signs such as weakness of the lower extremities, paresthesias, as well as neuropathies that interfere with normal function of the digestive tract and bladder can develop.

Steel related the KD to insignificant trauma generally involving the 3rd thoracic vertebra and the 2nd or 3rd lumbar vertebra predominantly observed in males. He also described five stages namely *initial insult*, characterized by hyperflexion of the spine and association to the trauma of variable type and severity, in addition to normal roentgenograms. The second stage or *post-traumatic period* was manifested by mild back pain without functional limitation. The third stage, *latent interval or state of relative well-being*, was characterized by progressive disability in the following week or months of the traumatic event, not incapacitated. In this period, variability in time from 4 weeks to 1 year has been described [2, 5, 7, 11, 14–18, 20–23]. Fourth stage or *recrudescent stage*, in this the patient presents localized, persistent back pain, tenderness, and tendency to peripheral irradiation. In the last stage or *terminal stage*, the patient develops permanent kyphotic deformity with or without progressive pressure on roots or spinal cord [2].

Neurological symptoms are usually absent in the early stages of the disease and when pain occurs in the thoracolumbar region this usually corresponds to the collapse of the vertebral body. In the advanced stages, the patient develops paresthesias, lower extremity weakness, and bowel/bladder disturbance [7]. Besides, the kyphotic deformity associated with osteoporotic vertebral fracture limits the functionality and has repercussions on the quality of life of the patient. In addition, it increases the mortality and incidence of fractures in adjacent bone structures [25, 26].

4. Risk factors in osteonecrosis

Numerous risk factors for AVN have been described including long-term glucocorticoid treatment, diabetes, alcoholism, osteoporosis, atherosclerosis, pancreatitis, cirrhosis, hypertriglyceridemia, vasculitis, acute trauma, radiotherapy, neoplasias, air or fat embolism, barotraumas hemoglobinopathies, such as sickle cell disease and infection.

4.1. Osteonecrosis and osteoporosis

As we know, osteoporosis is one of the metabolic disorders associated with compression fractures of the vertebrae. This affects the quality of life of patients, who develop progressive spinal deformities that deteriorate gait and balance [27], increasing the risk of fracture [8] and mortality [28]. As mentioned, one of the mechanisms most involved in post-traumatic vertebral collapse is ischemic necrosis frequently associated with IVC in osteoporotic spine fractures [29]. According to what has been reported in the literature, the IVC sign is not pathognomonic of KD and is common to observe in unstable osteoporotic CF [30]. Two stages in the evolution of the KD have been considered, although the pathophysiological mechanisms are not known with certainty. First, after the initial trauma, the vertebrae present partial or incomplete healing with consequent weakening. In this stage, the consolidation of an osteoporotic vertebral compression fracture is characterized by an active remodeling process. This includes resorption of necrotic bone and cartilaginous tissue, endochondral bone neoformation, new vessel formation and restoration of bone continuity in the fracture line. Likewise, zones of hypertrophic trabecular bone or areas with lack of bone repair can be observed; in addition, fragments of bone, cartilage and intervertebral disc can be sequestered in areas of dense fibrous and collagen tissue [31].

The second stage of the evolution of KD involved in this reparative failure could be impaired vertebral blood flow, herniation of nucleus pulposus into the vertebral body (Schmorl's nodes), and stress conditions in weakened vertebrae [3]. As it is known, the blood supply of each vertebra depends on branches of the corresponding segmental arteries, which nourish the vertebral body, the spinal canal and the posterior third (equatorial, metaphyseal and peripheral branches) [32, 33]. It was also reported that the supply of the ventral part of the vertebral body derives from the anterior central branches of the segmental arteries, whereas the supply of the dorsal part comes from the posterior central branches [34]. This distribution anatomy has been the explanation of the frequency of IVC in the anterosuperior and anteroinferior portions of the vertebral body. Generally, the involvement of the anterior third of the collapsed vertebral body represents the vascular watershed zone related to alterations in the blood supply [7, 35].

Although the pathogenesis of KD remains unknown, in addition to the ischemic process, the motion between the fracture ends has been considered a preponderant factor. Since Hasegawa's description of the intravertebral cleft with the presence of serous fluid, surrounded by smooth fibrocartilaginous tissue and absence of lining, as well as the motion between the ends of the fracture, the development of pseudarthrosis has been consistent [36]. This radiographically supported motion in the progressive disappearance of a radiolucent gas-like area and the appearance of an area of fluid-like signal intensity on MRI has suggested that the IVC results from a migration of intradiscal gas between the ends of the osteoporotic spine fractures [6, 37]. Then, this nonunion would correspond to the persistence of the radiolucent line of the cleft and the hypointense line on MRI.

It is even reported when confirming the occlusion of the segmental artery on magnetic resonance angiography and identifying the presence of thrombi in microscopic analysis. Then it was postulated that an insult in the segmental artery could lead to AVN of the vertebral body with the consequent nonunion. It was also suggested an analogy between the deficit of the blood flow and the mechanical insufficiency of the subchondral fracture in the AVN of the femoral head and the mechanisms of osteoporotic CF [38]. Occlusion of the predominantly anterior and peripheral metaphyseal arteries seems to be observed in fragments of the fracture. Necrotic cancellous bone and hyaline cartilage endplate with fracture callus, fibrosis, fibrin deposition and hemorrhage as changes in AVN have been described [38, 39]. Some observations have been made regarding these approaches. The collapse of the basivertebral foramen located between the two pedicles in osteoporotic CF could be involved in the ischemic process of the vertebral body. This foramen allows the passage of nerve branches, basivertebral veins and arteries derived from the segmental ones [33, 40–43].

4.2. Glucocorticoid treatment and osteonecrosis

Long-term glucocorticoid therapy is a predisposing factor that induces the deposition of intramedullary fat with secondary compression of intramedullary vascularity, development of fatty microemboli and microfractures associated with osteopenia [35]. Hypertrophy and hyperplasia of fat cells in the bone marrow [44], the consequent increase in intraosseous pressure, microcirculatory occlusion by emboli and/or thrombi and decreased blood flow are important elements in the pathophysiology of induced steroid-induced ON [45]. Also, these lead to a decrease in collagen synthesis and osteoblastic activity [46]. In experimental studies in animal models, it has been demonstrated in addition to the effect of lovastatin, lipid-lowering agent, on the differentiation of cells from bone marrow into adipocytes, the preventive action or reduction of steroid-induced ON [47]. Therefore, it was proposed that lovastatin suppresses steroid-induced adipogenesis, decreases the fat cell transcription factor PPARg2 expression and favors osteoblastic differentiation, as well as *in vivo* expression of *Cabf1/Runx2 genes* [47, 48]. Then, inhibition of hypertrophy and proliferation of bone marrow fat cells and the formation of emboli by the inhibitory action of hydroxymethylglutaryl-coenzyme A reductase decreases the possibility of microvascular occlusion [49, 50].

Several studies have reported the association of steroid use and decreased bone mineral density [51–53]. In this regard, long-term methylprednisolone treatment in immature pigs was used; it was observed that blood flow was reduced in endplates and cancellous bone in 61% of the cases and showed the correlation of ON with radiographic IVC [54]. This suggested that the reduction of blood supply could be a pathophysiological factor in glucocorticoid-induced ON and that its results did not vary depending on the projection expression (g/cm^2) or volumetric bone mineral density (g/cm^3) [54].

4.3. Vertebral osteonecrosis y pancreatitis

Few cases of vertebral intraosseous fat necrosis have been described [55, 56]. Its frequency is up to 0.8% and its main manifestations are multiple pathological fractures [56]. Pathophysiologically, the destruction of adipose tissue is a consequence of the lipolytic activity of the lipase released into the bloodstream [57]. Then, there is obstruction of the bone vascularity by drops of fat which leads to local intravascular coagulation and ON. In addition, intramedullary swelling and increased intraosseous pressure result from the release of prostaglandin E1 [58].

4.4. Type 1 Gaucher disease (GD1) and vertebral osteonecrosis

As is well known, Gaucher disease is a lysosomal storage disorder resulting from an autosomal recessive mutation in *GBA1 gene* that encodes acid β-glucosidase. Deficiency of this enzyme favors deposition of glucocerebroside in the lysosomes of mononuclear phagocytes from different organs including the skeleton [59, 60]. The main bone affections include osteopenia, fractures, and AVN [61, 62]. The clinical presentation may be silent as a spinal cord infarction due to asymptomatic obstruction of the vascularity of the bone marrow. Bone infarction is generally detected on MRI [63]. Although pathophysiological mechanisms have not been elucidated, various GBA1 genotypes associated with or without AVN have been reported [64].

Skeletal involvement in most patients with Gaucher disease is well known [59, 60, 65]. The main skeletal affections of this condition include AVN, osteopenia, and fractures [61, 62, 65]. Various authors refer to an incidence of 8–36.4% of spinal fractures in patients with GD1 [64, 66–70]. They proposed that anemia and decreased bone mineral density of the lumbar spine are strong risk factors for fractures and AVN [64].

It has been estimated that the risk of untreated AVN and GD1 is 22.8 per 1000 person-years of follow-up [71]. It has also been proposed that imiglucerase therapy reduces the presentation of AVN at 13.8 per 1000 years of follow-up [72]. The pathophysiology of AVN in GD1 is unknown, however, it is presumed to be associated with secondary spinal infarction likely to microvascular occlusion, visualized in MRI [63].

4.5. HIV and vertebral osteonecrosis

HIV infection has been reported as one of the factors associated with vertebral ON. In these patients, the use of corticosteroids, abuse of alcohol and tobacco, hypercoagulable states, treatment with antiretroviral drugs, lipodystrophy, and the use of megestrol acetate or testosterone have been reported as risk factors [73–83]. It is estimated that the incidence of ON in HIV-infected patients is 0.03–0.65 cases per 100 person-years [81, 84]. In all cases reported, the participation of one or more risk factors and multifocal involvement were considered [85, 86]. Likewise, HIV-infected patients without risk factors and ON have also been reported [87].

The prevalence of osteoporotic vertebral fractures in HIV-infected patients has been increasing [88]. Likewise, the association of ON in HIV-positive individuals has been reported [89]. In the literature, only two cases of vertebral ON in HIV-infected patients and treatment with highly active antiretroviral therapy (HAART) have been reported, which presented refractory pain and developed rapid progressive kyphotic deformity [90, 91]. Drugs such as tenofovir induce increased bone remodeling and demineralization favoring bone fragility and vertebral CF [92]. Also, therapy with protease inhibitors promotes fat infiltration of the bone marrowand increase of intraosseous pressure compromising vascular irrigation [93].

4.6. Sarcoidosis and vertebral osteonecrosis

Sarcoidosis is a systemic condition in which the involvement of the musculoskeletal system occurs in 5% of patients [94–97]. Although the spinal involvement in sarcoidosis is rare, about

30 patients in the literature have been reported. A patient with sarcoidosis discarded the possibility of osteoporotic vertebral collapse due to the shape and narrowing of the intravertebral groove, the involvement of the body and the posterior elements of the vertebra and lack of evidence of new bone formation in the collapsed body [19].

5. Radiographic characteristics

Radiographically, non-demonstrable evidence of a fracture in consecutive studies supports the diagnosis of KD [14]. However, it is important to perform the differential diagnosis between KD and nontraumatic or spontaneous vertebral ON associated with osteoporosis. Clinically, it should be emphasized that osteoporotic compression fractures are not associated with neurological symptomatology. On the other hand, chronic radiographic osteoporotic fractures are not associated with changes in signal intensity on MRI [35]. This contrasts with the variability in signal characteristics on MRI in KD [6, 98]. Usually, these appear with an increase in the signal on T1-weighted images and reduced signal on T2-weighted images. However, in both KD and spontaneous vertebral ON, a hyperintense linear area on MRI can be observed. This pattern of signal change has been referred "double line sign" and corresponds to the phenomenon of IVC. This describes the accumulation of gas in the vertebral body observed in X-ray studies (**Figure 1**). This sign has also been observed associated with malignancy and intraosseous disc herniation, so it should not be considered as pathognomonic of ON.

Another radiological sign associated with ON is the intravertebral fluid of the vertebral body. This appears as a well-circumscribed area of low signal intensity on T1-weighted MRI and high signal intensity on T2-weighted images [39, 99]. This characteristic is known as a sign of fluid. In this regard, it was reported the coexistence of air and fluid in the same vertebral body in 21.5% of the cases. It was observed a more severe vertebral collapse in those cases with only intravertebral air than in those with fluid with or without air [100].

6. Classification of Kümmel's disease

In an attempt to classify the alterations associated with KD, morphological analyses regarding the type, degree of deformity and severity of vertebral collapse with questionable clinical relevance in acute processes was proposed [101]. Later, was proposed a multidimensional scheme for the classification of VCF suggesting that it could have application in the selection of surgical treatment and follow-up of patients. This included six dimensions fracture morphometry, chronicity, repair, dynamic stability, rupture of intravertebral bone trabeculae or clefts, and involvement of the posterior cortex [102]. However, this has been considered complicated and without any correlation with a natural history of KD.

Then, another specific classification proposal for this disease is raised, dependent on the progression and sequential clinical changes of the same. For this scale, Stage I corresponded to vertebrae intact or with a loss of height of the anterior portion of the vertebral body of less than 20% and without IVC in plain X-ray films, with a small cleft and fluid sign on T2-weighted

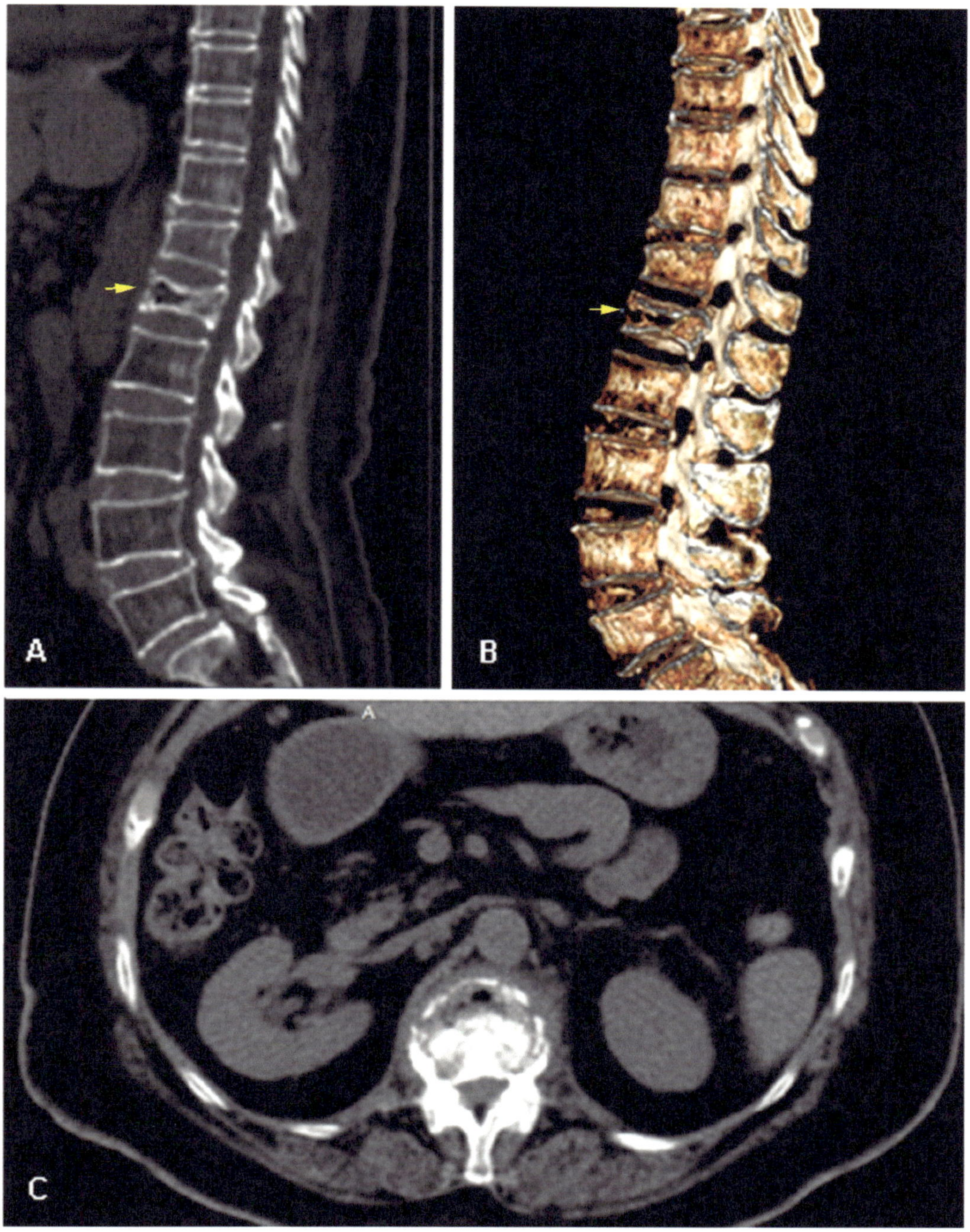

Figure 1. CT scan of the lumbar spine with compression fracture of L1 and intravertebral vacuum cleft (arrow). A Multiplanar reconstruction in sagittal, B volumetric reconstruction (3D), C axial plane.

MRI. In Stage II, loss of anterior body height would be more than 20% without an involvement of the posterior cortical, collapse of the vertebral body with dynamic mobility in the radiographs and presence of the cleft sign on MRI. Finally, in Stage III included the severe collapse of the vertebral body with dynamic mobility and rupture of the posterior cortical, as well as IVC with retropulsion of bone fragments and compression of the spinal cord. At this stage, the patients presented back pain, deformity and neurological deficit [103].

Also were reported three stages related to the pathogenesis of progression to delayed vertebral collapse. Stage 1 showed presence of intravertebral cleft, Stage 2 showed IVC plus intravertebral instability, and Stage 3 showed complete vertebral collapse [104]. We can summarize that the main application of these classification proposals has not only been to describe the evolution of osteoporotic CF, but also to evaluate the clinical efficacy and to determine the follow-up of different surgical procedures.

7. Histopathology

There are few reports in the literature describing the histopathological features of vertebral ON. The first autopsy material related to KD was presented in 1926 [105]. It was described the destruction of spongy bone tissue and the consequent collapse of the vertebral body. Later was reported the pathological examination of the wedge-shaped collapsed L2 vertebral body, atrophic changes in bone trabeculae and multiple hemorrhagic areas [106]. These findings were termed "multiple microscopic fractures" [107].

Afterward, four concentric zones in AVN were proposed. These were a central area of cell death, followed by ischemia, congestion, and a peripheral zone of normal tissue. Early, inflammatory cells, serosanguinolent fluid, without bacterial colonies have been described. Thus, both the ischemic and the congestive zone undergo repair changes being replaced by fibrous tissue or new bone [108, 109]. Likewise, an anatomopathological study of vertebral pseudarthrosis reported a whitish, smooth, fibrocartilage-like lining with scarce chondrocytes, and flattened fibroblasts. As well, the regions after the cleft presented granulation tissue and poor bone formation. The biochemical characteristics of the fluid contained in the cleft showed a similar composition to the blood plasma, except for the lower proportion of total proteins [36].

ON reported in histopathological analysis on biopsy material demonstrated consistent data of new bone formation, bone marrow fibrosis, and bone repair [7, 17, 18, 20, 22]. However, different advances have been proposed from the original approaches, "rarefying osteitis" of inflammatory origin, multiple trauma of bone and ligamentous structures with the formation of cracks and microhemorrhages that lead to ON.

Some studies have suggested the correlation of the sign of the fluid on MRI and the histopathological data of vertebral ON demonstrated by the presence of small necrotic bone fragments between a fibrous stroma. In this regard, it was showed the presence of ON, edema, and fibrosis associated with the sign of fluid and this was significantly related to the severity of the fracture [110].

It has been considered that in the early stages vertebral ON presents edema and exudate, whereas in the late stages air could be contained in the spaces formed by the sclerotic bone [39, 111]. Hence, possibly the changes were described from the intravertebral fluid to gas on MRI [100]. In addition to this proposal, it was reported that the sign of the fluid could be identified on MRI between 1 and 5 months, while the IVC could be noticed between 2 and 10 months after the fracture of the vertebra [112]. Subsequently, regenerative changes in more than 80% of cases occur, which are characterized by bone resorption, the formation of new bone and fibrosis. The still unstable collapse of the vertebra, the involvement of the spinal canal and neurological manifestations can be associated with these changes. However, some cases have been described with absence of unexplained regenerative histological changes [112].

Moreover, in those cases of vertebral body ON without vertebral collapse, empty lacunae, fatty necrosis with vacuolar degeneration and cell debris were described, suggesting necrosis of the bone marrow [113].

8. Differential diagnosis

The imaging characteristics described in vertebral ON such as sclerosis and calcification on computed tomography (CT) scan, hypointense images on T1 or hyperintense on T2, and non-reinforcement with Gadolinium (Gd) of the ischemic zone on MRI represent edema and necrosis. These changes could be confounded with other bone lesions such as the bone cyst, bone infarct, bone island, hemangioma, osteoblastoma, and osteoblastic metastatic tumor [113]. The literature reports cases of nontypical vertebral ON, on MRI, do not show low-intensity signal on T1 or double line sign on T2. In these cases, it has been suggested that the difference in the imaging findings could be due to the processes of ON and repair. Also, the vertebral bodies in these patients did not present collapse and the cortical intact was observed [113].

9. Treatment

As mentioned, the main symptom of delayed post-traumatic vertebral collapse is chronic back pain. This is usually localized, persistent, with a tendency to progression and irradiation to the peripheral nerve roots. Among conservative management protocols for back pain, the combination of exercise therapy and nonsteroidal anti-inflammatory drugs has been used with partially satisfactory results [114]. In addition to the medical aspects, psychosocial factors have been related to the pathophysiology of pain and response to treatment [115, 116]. Among this, anxiety, depression, notably distress and somatization have been associated, so strategies related to supportive psychotherapy, cognitive-behavioral methods and psychiatric medical treatments have been proposed in some cases [115, 117].

In some cases, teriparatide, an osteoanabolic agent frequently used in the treatment of osteoporosis, has been effective in promoting the reparative bone process and reducing pain [23, 118].

In the absence of neurological compromise and under the assumption of nonaffectation of the posterior cortical vertebral body has been suggested the conservative management of pain by analgesic drugs and bed rest [7]. It is now known that the incidence of vertebral compression following the conservative management of osteoporotic vertebral fractures reaches 14.8% at 1 month and 21.8% at 6 months [119]. However, when conservative management fails, minimally invasive procedures such as vertebroplasty or kyphoplasty are suggested to stabilize the fracture site, align the vertebral segment and consequently alleviate pain [23]. The first reports in the literature on the treatment of KD emphasize conservative management, whereas the latest information has demonstrated that patients can be treated successfully with surgery. The choice of surgical treatment has depended to a large extent upon three factors, the severity of the back pain, the degree of kyphotic deformity, and the neurologic deficit [5, 7]. The main objective of the surgery lies in the decompression of the neural elements and sagittal alignment, consequently, earlier ambulation is promoted [120].

Techniques such as percutaneous kyphoplasty (PKP) or percutaneous vertebroplasty (PVP) with polymethyl methacrylate (PMMA) have been used in patients with osteoporotic CF with and without IVC [10, 121–127]. It was reported on both types of surgical procedures to relieve pain and restore collapsed vertebral body immediately after surgery. However, they reported aggravation of vertebral collapse and kyphotic deformity within 2 years after surgery in those patients with IVC. This also conditioned an increase in back pain, suggesting that this progression was due to intravertebral instability [121]. Therefore, both PVP and PKP have been considered as noneffective procedures in chronic spinal compression or acute vertebral compression with posterior cortical rupture, suggesting surgical stabilization via fusion [128]. The response to a foreign body that can occur with the use of PMMA with extensive fibrosis that could induce micromotion and secondary instability should also be mentioned [129, 130]. In addition, the mass of PMMA could spontaneously migrate to extra vertebral sites such as the disc space or the anterior vertebral space [8, 131–133].

Likewise, the distribution pattern and proportion of bone cement required in PVP could be predicted according to the area of ischemic necrosis on MRI [134]. Also, taking into account the proportion of necrosis on MRI recently raised that this variable could allow selecting the type of surgical procedure vertebroplasty, kyphoplasty, or surgery. Those cases with IVC, as well as those that required a surgical procedure were those that presented a higher percentage of necrosis [119].

Another reported proposal was the management of the posttraumatic osteoporotic vertebral ON with balloon kyphoplasty. It was suggested that restoration of the vertebral body and correction of kyphotic deformation could be achieved in relation to the sufficient volume of cement used. In addition, cement injection was performed in middle to later stages of solidification in patients with a defect of the anterior wall of the vertebral body or supported by X-ray fluoroscopy and balloon expansion in posterior defects to avoid leakage of the same [127].

The anterior decompression via corporectomy and fusion with intervertebral tricortical graft [135, 136] or ceramic glass spacers [137], posterior decompression with pedicle subtraction osteotomy [138–140] or the combination of both approaches [139] have been proposed in several studies. In the previous decompression, the fusion can be achieved with a spacer and a plate with a screw and in the posterior approach by means of the placement of transpedicular screws and hooks [141]. Spinal fusion, however, has been associated with procedural complications and long surgical time.

Subsequently, the technique of posterior one-segmental fixation combined with vertebroplasty and posterior-shortening osteotomy showed satisfactory results regarding correction of deformity, pain relief and functional improvement in patients with KD [142]. However, due to short segment fixation failures [143], the use of long segments to reestablish sagittal alignment was proposed. In the cases, it was reported to remove the upper end plate of the affected vertebral body and the superior intervertebral disc during the transpedicular subtraction and disc osteotomy combined with long-segment fixation, which favored bone fusion [144]. The placement of cages and long-segment fixation in pedicle subtraction osteotomy and disc resection has been useful in thoracolumbar post-traumatic kyphosis [145].

Author details

Elizabeth Pérez Hernández*, Eulalio Elizalde Martínez and Juan Manuel Torres Fernández

*Address all correspondence to: elizabeth.perez@imss.gob.mx

UMAE de Traumatología, Ortopedia y Rehabilitación "Dr. Victorio de la Fuente Narváez," Instituto Mexicano del Seguro Social, Ciudad de México, México

References

[1] Kümmel H. Ueber die traumatischen Erkrankungen der. Deutsche Medizinische Wochenschrift. 1895;**21**:180-181

[2] Steel HH. Kümmell's disease. American Journal of Surgery. 1951;**81**(2):161-167

[3] Benedek TG, Nicholas JJ. Delayed traumatic vertebral body compression fracture; part II: Pathologic features. Seminars in Arthritis and Rheumatism. 1981;**10**(4):271-277. DOI: 10.1016/0049-0172(81)90004-4

[4] Rigler L. Kümmell's disease with report of a roentgenologically. American Journal of Roentgenology. 1931;**35**:749-753

[5] Ma R, Chow R, Shen FH. Kümmell's disease: Delayed post-traumatic osteonecrosis of the vertebral body. European Spine Journal. 2010;**19**(7):1065-1070. DOI: 10.1007/s00586-009-1205-4

[6] Maldague BE, Noel HM, Malghem JJ. The intravertebral vacuum cleft: A sign of ischemic vertebral collapse. Radiology. 1978;**129**(1):23-29

[7] Young WF, Brown D, Kendler A, Clements D. Delayed post-traumatic osteonecrosis of a vertebral body (Kümmell's disease). Acta Orthopaedica Belgica. 2002;**68**(1):13-19

[8] Kim DY, Lee SH, Jang JS, Chung SK, Lee HY. Intravertebral vacuum phenomenon in osteoporotic compression fracture: Report of 67 cases with quantitative evaluation of intravertebral instability. Journal of Neurosurgery. 2004;**100**(1 Suppl Spine):24-31

[9] Pappou IP, Papadopoulos EC, Swanson AN, Cammisa Jr FP, Girardi FP. Osteoporotic vertebral fractures and collapse with intravertebral vacuum sign (Kümmel's disease). Orthopedics. 2008;**31**(1):61-66

[10] Jang JS, Kim DY, Lee SH. Efficacy of percutaneous vertebroplasty in the treatment of intravertebral pseudarthrosis associated with noninfected avascular necrosis of the vertebral body. Spine (Philadelphia, PA 1976). 2003;**28**(14):1588-1592

[11] Van Eenenaam DP, el-Khoury GY. Delayed post-traumatic vertebral collapse (Kümmell's disease): Case report with serial radiographs, computed tomographic scans, and bone scans. Spine (Philadelphia, PA 1976). 1993;**18**(9):1236-1241

[12] Kim KT, Suk KS, Kim JM, Lee SH. Delayed vertebral collapse with neurological deficits secondary to osteoporosis. International Orthopaedics. 2003;**27**(2):65-69. DOI: 10.1007/s00264-002-0418-5

[13] Lee SH, Kim ES, Eoh W. Cement augmented anterior reconstruction with short posterior instrumentation: A less invasive surgical option for Kümmell's disease with cord compression. Journal of Clinical Neuroscience. 2011;**18**(4):509-514. DOI: 10.1016/j.jocn.2010.07.139

[14] Brower AC, Downey Jr EF. Kümmell disease: Report of a case with serial radiographs. Radiology. 1981;**141**(2):363-364. DOI: 10.1148/radiology.141.2.7291557

[15] Hermann G, Goldblatt J, Desnick RJ. Kümmell disease: Delayed collapse of the traumatised spine in a patient with Gaucher type 1 disease. The British Journal of Radiology. 1984;**57**(682):833-835. DOI: 10.1259/0007-1285-57-681-833

[16] Osterhouse MD, Kettner NW. Delayed posttraumatic vertebral collapse with intravertebral vacuum cleft. Journal of Manipulative & Physiological Therapeutics. 2002; **25**(4):270-275

[17] Kapoor V, Theruvil B, Foria V, Sampson M, Harley JM. Vertebral collapse in a 71-year-old woman. Clinical Orthopaedics and Related Research. 2004;**423**:291-298

[18] Maheshwari PR, Nagar AM, Prasad SS, Shah JR, Patkar DP. Avascular necrosis of spine: A rare appearance. Spine (Philadelphia, PA 1976). 2004;**29**(6):E119-E122

[19] Ito M, Motomiya M, Abumi K, Shirado O, Kotani Y, et al. Vertebral osteonecrosis associated with sarcoidosis. Case report. Journal of Neurosurgery Spine. 2005;**2**(2):222-225. DOI: 10.3171/spi.2005.2.2.0222

[20] Swartz K, Fee D. Kümmell's disease: A case report and literature review. Spine (Philadelphia, PA 1976). 2008;**33**(5):E152-E155. DOI: 10.1097/BRS.0b013e3181657f31

[21] Van der Schaaf I, Fransen H. Percutaneous vertebroplasty as treatment for Kümmell's disease. JBR-BTR. 2009;**92**(2):83-85

[22] Matzaroglou C, Georgiou CS, Assimakopoulos K, Saridis A, Khudiaev AT, et al. Kümmell' s disease: A rare spine entity in a young adult. Hellenic Journal of Nuclear Medicine. 2010; **13**(1):52-55

[23] Fabbriciani G, Pirro M, Floridi P, Callarelli L, Manfredelli MR, et al. Osteoanabolic therapy: A non-surgical option of treatment for Kümmell's disease?. Rheumatology International. 2012;**32**(5):1371-1374. DOI: 10.1007/s00296-010-1408-3

[24] Ranjan M, Mahadevan A, Prasad C, Sommana S, Susarla Krishna S. Kümmell's disease - uncommon or underreported disease: A clinicopathological account of a case and review of literature. Journal of Neurosciences in Rural Practice. 2013;**4**(4):439-442. DOI: 10.4103/0976-3147.120234

[25] Silverman SL, Minshall ME, Shen W, Harper KD, Xie S; Health-Related Quality of Life Subgroup of the Multiple Outcomes of Raloxifene Evaluation Study. The relationship of health-related quality of life to prevalent and incident vertebral fractures in postmenopausal women with osteoporosis: Results from the Multiple Outcomes of Raloxifene Evaluation Study. Arthritis and Rheumatism. 2001;**44**(11):2611-2619

[26] Hasserius R, Karlsson MK, Nilsson BE, Redlund-Johnell I, Johnell O; European Vertebral Osteoporosis Study. Prevalent vertebral deformities predict increased mortality and increased fracture rate in both men and women: A 10-year population-based study of 598 individuals from the Swedish cohort in the European Vertebral Osteoporosis Study. Osteoporos International. 2003;**14**(1):61-68. DOI: 10.1007/s00198-002-1316-9

[27] Gold DT. The clinical impact of vertebral fractures: Quality of life in women with osteoporosis. Bone. 1996;**18**(3 Suppl):185S-189S

[28] Kado DM, Huang MH, Karlamangla AS, Barrett-Connor E, Greendale GA. Hyperkyphotic posture predicts mortality in older community-dwelling men and women: A prospective study. Journal of the American Geriatrics Society. 2004;**52**(10):1662-1667. DOI: 10.1111/j.1532-5415.2004.52458.x

[29] McKiernan F, Faciszewski T. Intravertebral clefts in osteoporotic vertebral compression fractures. Arthritis and Rheumatism. 2003;**48**(5):1414-1419. DOI: 10.1002/art.10984

[30] McKiernan F, Jensen R, Faciszewski T. The dynamic mobility of vertebral compression fractures. Journal of Bone and Mineral Research. 2003;**18**(1):24-29. DOI: 10.1359/jbmr.2003.18.1.24

[31] Antonacci MD, Mody DR, Rutz K, Weilbaecher D, Heggeness MH. A histologic study of fractured human vertebral bodies. Journal of Spinal Disorders & Techniques. 2002;**15**(2) :118-126

[32] Crock HV, Yoshizawa H. The blood supply of the lumbar vertebral column. Clinical Orthopaedics and Related Research. 1976;**115**:6-21

[33] Ratcliffe JF. The arterial anatomy of the adult human lumbar vertebral body: A microarteriographic study. Journal of Anatomy. 1980;**131**(Pt 1):57-79

[34] Prakash, Prabhu LV, Saralaya VV, Pai MM, Ranade AV, et al. Vertebral body integrity: A review of various anatomical factors involved in the lumbar region. Osteoporos International. 2007;**18**(7):891-903. DOI: 10.1007/s00198-007-0373-5

[35] Chou LH, Knight RQ. Idiopathic avascular necrosis of a vertebral body. Case report and literature review. Spine (Philadelphia, PA 1976). 1997;**22**(16):1928-1932

[36] Hasegawa K, Homma T, Uchiyama S, Takahashi H. Vertebral pseudarthrosis in the osteoporotic spine. Spine (Philadelphia, PA 1976). 1988;**23**(20):2201-2206

[37] Lafforgue P, Chagnaud C, Daumen-Legré V, Daver L, Kasbarian M, et al. The intravertebral vacuum phenomenon ("vertebral osteonecrosis"). Migration of intradiscal gas in a fractured vertebral body?. Spine (Philadelphia, PA 1976). 1997;**22**(16):1885-1891

[38] Kim YC, Kim YH, Ha KY. Pathomechanism of intravertebral clefts in osteoporotic compression fractures of the spine. Spine Journal. 2014;**14**(4):659-666. DOI: 10.1016/j.spinee.2013.06.106

[39] Dupuy DE, Palmer WE, Rosenthal DI. Vertebral fluid collection associated with vertebral collapse. AJR American Journal of Roentgenology. 1996;**167**(6):1535-1538

[40] Wang C, Fan S, Liu J, Suyou L, Shan Z, et al. Basivertebral foramen could be connected with intravertebral cleft: A potential risk factor of cement leakage in percutaneous kyphoplasty. Spine Journal. 2014;**14**(8):1551-1558. DOI: 10.1016/j.spinee.2013.09.025

[41] Antonacci MD, Mody DR, Heggeness MH. Innervation of the human vertebral body: A histologic study. Journal of Spinal Disorders. 1998;**11**(6):526-531

[42] Fras C, Kravetz P, Mody DR, Heggeness MH. Substance P-containing nerves within the human vertebral body. An immunohistochemical study of the basivertebral nerve. Spine Journal. 2003;**3**(1):63-67

[43] Crock HV, Yoshizawa H, Kame SK. Observations on the venous drainage of the human vertebral body. The Journal of Bone and Joint Surgery. 1973;**55**(3):528-533

[44] Wang GJ, Cui Q, Balian G. The Nicolas Andry award. The pathogenesis and prevention of steroid-induced osteonecrosis. Clinical Orthopaedics and Related Research. 2000;**370**:295-310

[45] Koo KH, Dussault RG, Kaplan PA, Ahn IO, Kim R, et al. Fatty marrow conversion of the proximal femoral metaphysis in osteonecrotic hips. Clinical Orthopaedics and Related Research. 1999;**361**:159-167

[46] Yamamoto T, Hirano K, Tsutsui H, Sugioka Y, Sueishi K. Corticosteroid enhances the experimental induction of osteonecrosis in rabbits with Shwartzman reaction. Clinical Orthopaedics and Related Research. 1995;**316**:235-243

[47] Pengde K, Fuxing P, Bin S, Jing Y, Jingqiu C. Lovastatin inhibits adipogenesis and prevents osteonecrosis in steroid-treated rabbits. Joint Bone Spine. 2008;**75**(6):696-701. DOI: 10.1016/j.jbspin.2007.12.008

[48] Li X, Cui Q, Kao C, Wang GJ, Balian. Lovastatin inhibits adipogenic and stimulates osteogenic differentiation by suppressing PPARgamma2 and increasing Cbfa1/Runx2 expression in bone marrow mesenchymal cell cultures. Bone. 2003;**33**(4):652-659

[49] Wang GJ, Chung KC, Shen WJ. Lipid clearing agents in steroid-induced osteoporosis. Journal of the Formosan Medical Association. 1995;**94**(10):589-592

[50] Wang GJ. Pathogenesis of steroid-induced avascular necrosis and its response to lipid clearing agents. In: Hirohata K, Mizuno K, Matsubara T, editors. Trends in Research and Treatment of Joint Diseases. Tokyo: Springer-Verlag; 1992. pp. 59-71. DOI: 10.1007/978-4-431-68192-2_8

[51] Fritz PC, Ward WE, Atkinson SA, Tenenbaum HC. Tamoxifen attenuates the effects of exogenous glucocorticoid on bone formation and growth in piglets. Endocrinology. 1998; **139**(8):3399-3403

[52] Weinstein RS, Jilka RL, Parfitt AM, Manolagas SC. Inhibition of osteoblastogenesis and promotion of apoptosis of osteoblasts and osteocytes by glucocorticoids. Potential mechanisms of their deleterious effects on bone. Journal of Clinical Investigation. 1998; **102**(2):274-282

[53] Julian BA, Laskow DA, Dubovsky J, Dubovsky EV, Curtis JJ, et al. Rapid loss of vertebral mineral density after renal transplantation. The New England Journal of Medicine. 1991;**325**(8):544-550

[54] Drescher W, Li H, Qvesel D, Jensen SD, Flo C, et al. Vertebral blood flow and bone mineral density during long-term corticosteroid treatment: An experimental study in immature pigs. Spine (Philadelphia, PA 1976). 2000;**25**(23):3021-3025

[55] Allen BL, Jinkins WJ. Vertebral osteonecrosis associated with pancreatitis in child. A case report. Journal of Bone and Joint Surgery. 1978;**60**(7):985-987

[56] Sigmundsson FG, Andersen PB, Schroeder HD, Thomsen K. Vertebral osteonecrosis associated with pancreatitis in a woman with pancreas divisum. A case report. Journal of Bone and Joint Surgery. 2004;**86-A**(11):2504-2508

[57] Jones Jr JP. Fat embolism and osteonecrosis. Orthopedic Clinics of North America. 1985;**16**(4):595-633

[58] Rittenberg GM, Korn JH, Schabel SI, Stalheim R. Rapid osteolysis in pancreatic carcinoma. The Western Journal of Medicine. 1981;**135**(5):408-410

[59] Grabowski G, Kolodny E, Weinreb N, Rosenbloom B, Prakash-Cheng A, et al. Gaucher disease: Phenotypic and genetic variation. In: Scriver C, Beaudet A, Valle D, Sly W, editors. The Online Metabolic and Molecular Basis of Inherited Metabolic Disease. New York: McGraw-Hill Publishers; 2010. DOI: 10.1036/ommbid.177

[60] Charrow J, Andersson HC, Kaplan P, Kolodny EH, Mistry P, et al. The Gaucher registry: Demographics and disease characteristics of 1698 patients with Gaucher disease. Archives of Internal Medicine. 2000;**160**(18):2835-2843

[61] Stirnemann J, Belmatoug N, Vincent C, Fain O, Fantin B, et al. Bone events and evolution of biologic markers in Gaucher disease before and during treatment. Arthritis Research & Therapy. 2010;**12**(4):R156. DOI: 10.1186/ar3111

[62] Deegan PB, Pavlova E, Tindall J, Stein PE, Bearcroft P, et al. Osseous manifestations of adult Gaucher disease in the era of enzyme replacement therapy. Medicine (Baltimore). 2011;**90**(1):52-60. DOI: 10.1097/MD.0b013e3182057be4

[63] Lutsky KF, Tejwani NC. Orthopaedic manifestations of Gaucher disease. Bulletin of the Hospital for Joint Diseases. 2007;**65**(1):37-42

[64] Khan A, Hangartner T, Weinreb NJ, Taylor JS, Mistry PK. Risk factors for fractures and avascular osteonecrosis in type 1 Gaucher disease: A study from the International Collaborative Gaucher Group (ICGG) Gaucher Registry. Journal of Bone and Mineral Research. 2012;**27**(8):1839-1848. DOI: 10.1002/jbmr.1680

[65] Wenstrup RJ, Roca-Espiau M, Weinreb NJ, Bembi B. Skeletal aspects of Gaucher disease: A review. The British Journal of Radiology. 2002;**75**(Suppl 1):A2-A12. DOI: 10.1259/bjr.75.suppl_1.750002

[66] Zimran A, Kay A, Gelbart T, Garver P, Thurston D, et al. Gaucher disease. Clinical, laboratory, radiologic, and genetic features of 53 patients. Medicine (Baltimore). 1992;**71**(6):337-353

[67] Stirnemann J. Clinical study of the French cohort of Gaucher disease patients. La Revue De Medecine **Interne**. 2006;**27**(Suppl 1):S18-S21

[68] Belmatoug N, Billette de Villemeur T. Skeletal response to enzyme replacement therapy for type 1 Gaucher disease: A preliminary report of the French experience. Seminars in Hematology. 1995;**32**(Suppl 1):33-38

[69] Katz K, Sabato S, Horev G, Cohen IJ, Yosipovitch Z. Spinal involvement in children and adolescents with Gaucher disease. Spine (Philadelphia, PA 1976). 1993;**18**(3):332-335

[70] Javier RM, Moser T, Dietemann JL, Sparsa L, Natarajan-Ame S, et al. Multiple vertebral osteonecrosis. Joint Bone Spine. 2008;**75**(3):341-344. DOI: 10.1016/j.jbspin.2007.05.010

[71] Yeh M, Weinreb N, Deegan P, Vellodi A, Cole J, et al. Avascular necrosis in untreated patients with type 1 Gaucher disease. Molecular Genetics and Metabolism. 2009;**98**:62

[72] Mistry PK, Deegan P, Vellodi A, Cole JA, Yeh M, et al. Timing of initiation of enzyme replacement therapy after diagnosis of type 1 Gaucher disease: Effect on incidence of avascular necrosis. British Journal of Haematology. 2009;**147**(4):561-570. DOI: 10.1111/j.1365-2141.2009.07872.x

[73] Aguiar De Aragao P, Lemos RB, Aquino MZ, Souza Marques HH. Hyperlipidaemia a risk factor for femoral head osteonecrosis (Legg-Calv -Perthes-like disease) in children with AIDS: Case report. Brazilian Journal of Infectious Diseases. 2002;**6**:142-145

[74] Allison GT, Bostrom MP, Glesby MJ. Osteonecrosis in HIV disease: Epidemiology, etiologies, and clinical management. AIDS. 2003;**17**(1):1-9. DOI: 10.1097/01.aids.0000042940.55529.93

[75] Glesby MJ, Hoover DR, Vaamonde CM. Osteonecrosis in patients infected with human immunodeficiency virus: A case-control study. The Journal of Infectious Diseases. 2001;**184**:519-523. DOI: 10.1086/322779

[76] Hasse B, Ledergerber B, Egger M, Flepp M, Bachmann S, et al; Swiss HIV Cohort Study. Antiretroviral treatment and osteonecrosis in patients of the Swiss HIV Cohort Study: A nested case-control study. AIDS Research and Human Retroviruses. 2004;**20**(9):909-915. DOI: 10.1089/aid.2004.20.909

[77] Martin K, Lawson-Ayayi S, Miremont-Salamé G, Blaizeau MJ, Balestre E, et al; Groupe d'Epidémiologie Clinique du SIDA en Aquitaine. Symptomatic bone disorders in HIV-infected patients: Incidence in the Aquitaine cohort (1999-2002). HIV Medicine. 2004;**5**(6):421-426. DOI: 10.1111/j.1468-1293.2004.00247.x

[78] Miller KD, Masur H, Jones EC, Joe GO, Rick ME, et al. High prevalence of osteonecrosis of the femoral head in HIV-infected adults. Annals of Internal Medicine. 2002;**137**(1):17-25

[79] Molia AC, Strady C, Rouger C, Beguinot IM, Berger JL, et al. Osteonecrosis in six HIV-infected patients receiving highly active antiretroviral therapy. Annals of Pharmacotherapy. 2004;**38**(12):2050-2054. DOI: 10.1345/aph.1E154

[80] Blacksin MF, Kloser PC, Simon J. Avascular necrosis of bone in human immunodeficiency virus infected patients. Clinical Imaging. 1999;**23**(5):314-318

[81] Scribner AN, Troia-Cancio PV, Cox BA, Marcantonio D, Hamid F, et al. Osteonecrosis in HIV: A case-control study. Journal of Acquired Immune Deficiency Syndromes. 2000;**25** (1):19-25

[82] Valencia ME, Barreiro P, Soriano V, Blanco F, Moreno V, et al. Avascular necrosis in HIV-infected patients receiving antiretroviral treatment: Study of seven cases. HIV Clinical Trials. 2003;**4**(2):132-136. DOI: 10.1310/hct.2003.4.2.008

[83] Koller E, Mann M, Malozowski S, Bacsanyi J, Gibert C. Aseptic necrosis in HIV seropositive patients: A possible etiologic role for megestrol acetate. AIDS Patient Care STDS. 2000;**14**(8):405-410. DOI: 10.1089/108729100416614

[84] Gutiérrez F, Padilla S, Ortega E, García JA, Flores J, et al. Avascular necrosis of the bone in HIV-infected patients: Incidence and associated factors. AIDS. 2002;**16**(3):481-483

[85] Gutiérrez F, Padilla S, Masiá M, Flores J, Boix V, et al; HIV-related Osteonecrosis Study Group. Osteonecrosis in patients infected with HIV: Clinical epidemiology and natural history in a large case series from Spain. Journal of Acquired Immune Deficiency Syndromes. 2006;**42**(5):650. DOI: 10.1097/01.qai.0000225012.53568.20

[86] González García A, Sifuentes Giraldo WA, Blázquez Cañamero MÁ, Ahijón Lana M, Navas Elorza E, et al. Multifocal osteonecrosis associated with human immunodeficiency virus infection. Reumatologia Clinica. 2012;**8**(6):361-364. DOI: 10.1016/j.reuma.2012.01.008

[87] Monier P, McKown K, Bronze MS. Osteonecrosis complicating highly active antiretroviral therapy in patients infected with human immunodeficiency virus. Clinical Infectious Diseases. 2000;**31**(6):1488-1492. DOI: 10.1086/317503

[88] Young B, Dao CN, Buchacz K, Baker R, Brooks JT; HIV Outpatient Study (HOPS) Investigators. Increased rates of bone fracture among HIV-infected persons in the HIV

Outpatient Study (HOPS) compared with the US general population, 2000-2006. Clinical Infectious Diseases. 2011;**52**(8):1061-1068. DOI: 10.1093/cid/ciq242

[89] Fessel WJ, Chau Q, Leong D. Association of osteonecrosis and osteoporosis in HIV-1-infected patients. AIDS. 2011;**25**(15):1877-1880. DOI: 10.1097/QAD.0b013e32834af637

[90] Sifuentes Giraldo WA, Blázquez Cañamero M, Navas Elorza E, Gallego Rivera I, Vázquez Díaz M. Concomitant presentation of multiple vertebral and peripheral osteonecrosis in a HIV-infected patient. Joint Bone Spine. 2012;**79**(3):332-334. DOI: 10.1016/j.jbspin.2011.12.002

[91] Sifuentes Giraldo WA, Macía Villa CC, Rodríguez-Navarro CQ, Vázquez Díaz M. Vertebral osteonecrosis in an HIV-infected patient. Antiviral Therapy. 2012;**17**(8):1627-1630. DOI: 10.3851/IMP2262

[92] Guo FP, Yu XB, Luo L, Han Y, Qiu ZF, et al. The impact of highly active antiretroviral therapy on bone mineral density in human immunodeficiency virus infected patients. Zhonghua Nei Ke Za Zhi. 2010;**49**(8):649-652

[93] Porsch M, König DP, Popken F. Possible complication of HIV therapy. Protease inhibitor-induced femur head necrosis. MMW Fortschritte Der Medizin. 2001;**143**(Suppl 1):90-91

[94] Fallon MD, Perry 3rd HM, Teitelbaum SL. Skeletal sarcoidosis with osteopenia. Metabolic Bone Disease & Related Research. 1981;**3**(3):171-174

[95] Resnik CS, Young JW, Aisner SC, Levine A. Case report 594: Osseous sarcoidosis (osteolytic) of lumbar spine and pelvis. Skeletal Radiology. 1990;**19**(1):79-81

[96] Rúa-Figueroa I, Gantes MA, Erausquin C, Mhaidli H, Montesdeoca A. Vertebral sarcoidosis: Clinical and imaging findings. Seminars in Arthritis and Rheumatism. 2002;**31**(5): 346-352

[97] Shaikh S, Soubani AO, Rumore P, Cantos E, Jelveh Z. Lytic osseous destruction in vertebral sarcoidosis. New York State Journal of Medicine. 1992;**92**(5):213-214

[98] Chevalier X, Wrona N, Avouac B, Larget-Piet B. Thigh pain and multiple vertebral osteonecroses: Value of magnetic resonance imaging. Journal of Rheumatology. 1991;**18**(10): 1627-1630

[99] Malghem J, Maldague B, Labaisse MA, Dooms G, Duprez T, et al. Intravertebral vacuum cleft: Changes in content after supine positioning. Radiology. 1993;**187**(2):483-487

[100] Yu CW, Hsu CY, Shih TT, Chen BB, Fu CJ. Vertebral osteonecrosis: MR imaging findings and related changes on adjacent levels. AJNR American Journal of Neuroradiology. 2007;**28**(1):42-47

[101] Eastell R, Cedel SL, Wahner HW, Riggs BL, Melton 3rd LJ. Classification of vertebral fractures. Journal of Bone and Mineral Research. 1991;**6**(3):207-215

[102] Faciszewski T, McKiernan F. Calling all vertebral fractures classification of vertebral compression fractures: A consensus for comparison of treatment and outcome. Journal of Bone and Mineral Research. 2002;**17**(2):185-191. DOI: 10.1359/jbmr.2002.17.2.185

[103] Li KC, †Wong TU, Kung FC, Li A, Hsieh CH. Staging of Kümmell's disease. Musculoskeletal Research. 2004;**8**(1):43-55. DOI: 10.1142/S0218957704001181

[104] Ito Y, Hasegawa Y, Toda K, Nakahara S. Pathogenesis and diagnosis of delayed vertebral collapse resulting from osteoporotic spinal fracture. Spine Journal. 2002;**2**(2):101-106

[105] Schmorl G, Junghanns H. The Human Spine in Health and Disease. 2nd ed. New York: Grune & Stratton; 1971. pp. 268-296

[106] Cardis J, Walker GF, Olver RH. Kümmell's disease. British Journal of Surgery. 1928;**15** (616):25

[107] Kux E. Zur Histopathologie der posttraumatischen (Kümmellschen) Wirbelerkrankung. Archiv für orthopädische und Unfall-Chirurgie, mit besonderer Berücksichtigung der Frakturenlehre und der orthopädisch-chirurgischen Technik. 1933;**34**:18-23

[108] Sweet DE, Madewell JE, Resnick DK, Niwayama E. Pathogenesis of osteonecrosis. In: Diagnosis of Bone and Joint Disorders. Philadelphia: Saunders; 1981. pp. 2780-2831

[109] Naul LG, Peet GJ, Maupin WB. Avascular necrosis of the vertebral body: MR imaging. Radiology. 1989;**172**(1):219-222

[110] Baur A, Stäbler A, Arbogast S, Duerr HR, Bartl R, et al. Acute osteoporotic and neoplastic vertebral compression fractures: Fluid sign at MR imaging. Radiology. 2002;**225**(3):730-735. DOI: 10.1148/radiol.2253011413

[111] Sugano N, Masuhara K, Nakamura N, Ochi T, Hirooka A, et al. MRI of early osteonecrosis of the femoral head after transcervical fracture. The Journal of Bone and Joint Surgery. British Volume. 1996;**78**(2):253-257

[112] Lin CL, Lin RM, Huang KY, Yan JJ, Yan YS. MRI fluid sign is reliable in correlation with osteonecrosis after vertebral fractures: A histopathologic study. European Spine Journal. 2013;**22**(7):1617-1623. DOI: 10.1007/s00586-012-2618-z

[113] Murakami H, Kawahara N, Gabata T, Nambu K, Tomita K. Vertebral body osteonecrosis without vertebral collapse. Spine (Philadelphia, PA 1976). 2003;**28**(16):E323-E328

[114] Van Tulder MW, Koes BW, Bouter LM. Conservative treatment of acute and chronic nonspecific low back pain. A systematic review of randomized controlled trials of the most common interventions. Spine (Philadelphia, PA 1976). 1997;**22**(18):2128-2156

[115] Moore JE. Chronic low back pain and psychosocial issues. Physical Medicine and Rehabilitation Clinics of North America. 2010;**21**(4):801-815. DOI: 10.1016/j.pmr.2010.06.005

[116] Pincus T, Burton AK, Vogel S, Field AP. A systematic review of psychological factors as predictors of chronicity/disability in prospective cohorts of low back pain. Spine (Philadelphia, PA 1976). 2002;**27**(5):E109-E120

[117] Staiger TO, Gaster B, Sullivan MD, Deyo RA. Systematic review of antidepressants in the treatment of chronic low back pain. Spine (Philadelphia, PA 1976). 2003;**28**(22):2540-2545. DOI: 10.1097/01.BRS.0000092372.73527.BA

[118] Neer RM, Arnaud CD, Zanchetta JR, Prince R, Gaich GA, et al. Effect of parathyroid hormone (1-34) on fractures and bone mineral density in postmenopausal women with osteoporosis. New England Journal of Medicine. 2001;**344**(19):1434-1441. DOI: 10.1056/NEJM200105103441904

[119] Lee JM, Lee YS, Kim YB, Park SW, Kang DH, et al. What effects does necrotic area of Contrast-Enhanced MRI in osteoporotic vertebral fracture have on further compression and clinical outcome? Journal of Korean Neurosurgical Society. 2017;**60**(2):181-188. DOI: 10.3340/jkns.2016.0707.015

[120] Li KC, Li AF, Hsieh CH, Liao TH, Chen CH. Another option to treat Kümmell's disease with cord compression. European Spine Journal. 2007;**16**(9):1479-1487. DOI: 10.1007/s00586-006-0094-z

[121] Fang X, Yu F, Fu S, Song H. Intravertebral clefts in osteoporotic compression fractures of the spine: Incidence, characteristics, and therapeutic efficacy. International Journal of Clinical and Experimental Medicine. 2015;**8**(9):16960-16968

[122] Wu MH, Huang TJ, Cheng CC, Li YY, Hsu RW. Role of the supine lateral radiograph of the spine in vertebroplasty for osteoporotic vertebral compression fracture: A prospective study. BMC Musculoskeletal Disorder. 2010;**11**:164. DOI: 10.1186/1471-2474-11-164

[123] Kim YJ, Lee JW, Kim KJ, Chung SK, Kim HJ, et al. Percutaneous vertebroplasty for intravertebral cleft: Analysis of therapeutic effects and outcome predictors. Skeletal Radiology. 2010;**39**(8):757-766. DOI: 10.1007/s00256-009-0866-8

[124] Lane JI, Maus TP, Wald JT, Thielen KR, Bobra S, et al. Intravertebral clefts opacified during vertebroplasty: Pathogenesis, technical implications, and prognostic significance. AJNR American Journal of Neuroradiology. 2002;**23**(10):1642-1646

[125] Becker S, Tuschel A, Chavanne A, Meissner J, Ogon M. Balloon kyphoplasty for vertebra plana with or without osteonecrosis. Journal of Orthopaedic Surgery (Hong Kong). 2008;**16**(1):14-19. DOI: 10.1177/230949900801600104

[126] Heo DH, Choi JH, Kim MK, Choi HC, Jeong JH, et al. Therapeutic efficacy of vertebroplasty in osteoporotic vertebral compression fractures with avascular osteonecrosis: A minimum 2-year follow-up study. Spine (Philadelphia, PA 1976). 2012;**37**(7):E423-E429. DOI: 10.1097/BRS.0b013e318238f29a

[127] Wang G, Yang H, Meng B, Zhu X, Zou J, et al. Post-traumatic osteoporotic vertebral osteonecrosis treated using balloon kyphoplasty. Journal of Clinical Neuroscience. 2011;**18**(5):664-668. DOI: 10.1016/j.jocn.2010.09.014

[128] Zhang GQ, Gao YZ, Zheng J, Luo JP, Tang C, et al. Posterior decompression and short segmental pedicle screw fixation combined with vertebroplasty for Kümmell's disease with neurological deficits. Experimental and Therapeutic Medicine. 2013;**5**(2):517-522. DOI: 10.3892/etm.2012.833

[129] Lewis G. Properties of acrylic bone cement: State of the art review. Journal of Biomedical Materials Research. 1997;**38**(2):155-182

[130] Huang KY, Yan JJ, Lin RM. Histopathologic findings of retrieved specimens of vertebroplasty with polymethylmethacrylate cement: Case control study. Spine (Philadelphia, PA 1976). 2005;**30**(19):E585-E588

[131] Cho SM, Heo DH, Cho YJ. Spontaneous migration of a polymethylmethacrylate mass after vertebroplasty in osteoporotic lumbar compression fracture with avascular osteonecrosis: A case report. Joint Bone Spine. 2011;**78**(1):98-99. DOI: 10.1016/j.jbspin.2010.08.016

[132] Wang HS, Kim HS, Ju CI, Kim SW. Delayed bone cement displacement following balloon kyphoplasty. Journal of Korean Neurosurgical Society. 2008;**43**(4):212-214. DOI: 10.3340/jkns.2008.43.4.212

[133] Ha KY, Lee JS, Kim KW, Chon JS. Percutaneous vertebroplasty for vertebral compression fractures with and without intravertebral clefts. The Journal of Bone and Joint Surgery. 2006;**88**(5):629-633. DOI: 10.1302/0301-620X.88B5.17345

[134] Oka M, Matsusako M, Kobayashi N, Uemura A, Numaguchi Y. Intravertebral cleft sign on fat-suppressed contrast-enhanced MR: Correlation with cement distribution pattern on percutaneous vertebroplasty. Academic Radiology. 2005;**12**(8):992-999. DOI: 10.1016/j.acra.2005.05.003

[135] Kanayama M, Ishida T, Hashimoto T, Shigenobu K, Togawa D, et al. Role of major spine surgery using Kaneda anterior instrumentation for osteoporotic vertebral collapse. Journal of Spinal Disorders & Techniques. 2010;**23**(1):53-56. DOI: 10.1097/BSD.0b013e318193e3a5

[136] Hasegawa K, Homma T, Uchiyama S, Takahashi HE. Osteosynthesis without instrumentation for vertebral pseudarthrosis in the osteoporotic spine. The Journal of Bone and Joint Surgery. 1997;**79**(3):452-456

[137] Kaneda K, Asano S, Hashimoto T, Satoh S, Fujiya M. The treatment of osteoporotic-posttraumatic vertebral collapse using the Kaneda device and a bioactive ceramic vertebral prosthesis. Spine (Philadelphia, PA 1976). 1992;**17**(8 Suppl)):S295-S303

[138] Mochida J, Toh E, Chiba M, Nishimura K. Treatment of osteoporotic late collapse of a vertebral body of thoracic and lumbar spine. Journal of Spinal Disorders. 2001;**14**(5):393-398

[139] Suk SI, Kim JH, Lee SM, Chung ER, Lee JH. Anterior-posterior surgery versus posterior closing wedge osteotomy in posttraumatic kyphosis with neurologic compromised osteoporotic fracture. Spine (Philadelphia, PA 1976). 2003;**28**(18):2170-2175. DOI: 10.1097/01.BRS.0000090889.45158.5A

[140] Saita K, Hoshino Y, Kikkawa I, Nakamura H. Posterior spinal shortening for paraplegia after vertebral collapse caused by osteoporosis. Spine (Philadelphia, PA 1976). 2000;**25**(21):2832-2835

[141] Kim HS, Heo DW. Percutaneous pedicle screw fixation with polymethylmethacrylate augmentation for the treatment of thoracolumbar intravertebral pseudoarthrosis

associated with kümmell's osteonecrosis. BioMed Research International. 2016;**2016:**3878063. DOI: 10.1155/2016/3878063

[142] Long HQ, Wan Y, Zhang X, Liu SY, Li FB. Two kinds of posterior approach for Kvmmell's disease after osteoporotic thoracolumbar fracture. Chinese Journal of Traumatology. 2009;**12**(3):142-147

[143] Matsuyama Y, Goto M, Yoshihara H, Tsuji T, Sakai Y, et al. Vertebral reconstruction with biodegradable calcium phosphate cement in the treatment of osteoporotic vertebral compression fracture using instrumentation. Journal of Spinal Disorders & Techniques. 2004;**17**(4):291-296

[144] Zhang X, Hu W, Yu J, Wang Z, Wang Y. An effective rreatment option for kümmell disease with neurological eficits: Modified transpedicular subtraction and disc osteotomy combined with Long-Segment fixation. Spine (Philadelphia, PA 1976). 2016;**41**(15):E923-E930. DOI: 10.1097/BRS.0000000000001467

[145] Hu W, Wang B, Run H, Zhang X, Wang Y. Pedicle subtraction osteotomy and disc resection with cage placement in post-traumatic thoracolumbar kyphosis, a retrospective study. Journal of Orthopaedic Surgery and Research. 2016;**11**(1):112. DOI: 10.1186/s13018-016-0447-1

Section 2

Dentistry

Chapter 4

Osteonecrosis of the Jaws. Prevalence, Risk Factors and Role of Microbiota and Inflammation in a Population of Spain

Mario Pérez-Sayáns, Carmen Vidal-Real,
José M. Suárez-Peñaranda and Abel García-García

Additional information is available at the end of the chapter

http://dx.doi.org/10.5772/intechopen.69315

Abstract

Introduction: The purpose of this article is to determine the prevalence of ONJ in patients who have undergone intravenous bisphosphonate therapy, and relate the risk factors described (including Actinomices); indeed, to establish a protocol to reduce the risk of developing ONJ and to evaluate the evolution of the patient according to the sample's antibiogram.

Results: The prevalence of ONJ was 12.9%. Most of the non-diabetic patients did not develop ONJ (92.3%) ($p = 0.048$). In regards to the periodontal state, 94.3% of patients without periodontal problems did not develop ONJ ($p = 0.001$). Almost 50% of the necrosis were unifocal and located on the mandible ($p < 0.001$). The number of affected patients and the aggressiveness of the disease increased significantly three years after starting treatment ($p < 0.001$). 87.5% of biopsies showed the presence of Actinomyces. The inflammatory response was very variable, ranging from absent to intense but it increased with age ($p = 0.005$). The combination of amoxicillin with clavulanic acid showed good sensitivity in the majority of patients (82.6%).

Conclusions: As the etiology of ONJ remains unknown, it is essential to prioritize prevention while assessing the risk factors.

Keywords: osteonecrosis, bisphosphonates, prevalence, risk factors, microbiota, inflammation, actinomyces

1. Osteonecrosis of the jaws

1.1. History

The term osteonecrosis dates back to the 1950s, when a series of cancer patients who underwent radiotherapy developed bone lesions on the jaws following the treatment [1–3]. This treatment, which is currently resulting in many complications on an oral level, makes it very hard to cure infections that are sometimes inevitable for these patients, since ischemia takes place on the jaws.

Some years later, the first article appeared citing a periapical lesion following arsenic infiltration for canal treatment. Arsenic was used as a therapeutic agent and as poison in Ancient Greek and Roman times [4]. It was also used as an agent during dental history for pulp devitalization, when anesthetics did not exist. Due to its ability to destroy cells in surrounding tissues, the use of arsenic trioxide in vital pulpectomy has been dropped progressively [5]. Dumlu's article (2007) described a case of jaw necrosis in a young patient following tooth extraction of a first failed molar after arsenic treatment of the canals [6]. Toxavit, another devitalizing agent, has also been related to bone necrosis. In any case, both agents are currently obsolete for these dental treatments [7, 8].

Another one of the causes mentioned in the history of osteonecrosis is the untreated intracapsular fracture, after several months, the described clinical symptoms were pain in the temporal-jaw articulation in the affected side and the limitation in opening the jaw. On a radiographic level, the condylar head is usually eroded and irregular [9].

Back in 1982, the first cases of osteonecrosis of the jaw in toothless patients by chemotherapy treatment were published. Specifically, the article considered the origin was a lesion on the mucosa due to a trauma caused by removable prosthesis.

The cases of aseptic osteonecrosis after jaw osteotomy following orthognathic surgeries have also been described in the literature; they have been related mostly to a complication following a surgical error [10].

In 2002, a clinical case of osteonecrosis of the jaws due to chemotherapy in a patient with myelogenous leukemia was published [11]; and, a year later, the current term bisphosphonates-related osteonecrosis of the jaws was branded (BRONJ) [12].

Despite the osteonecrosis of the jaws was exclusively related to the mouth, some rare cases in the external ear, the hip, the tibia and the femur have been documented [13, 14].

1.2. Definition

The concept of osteonecrosis of the jaws was introduced in 2003 when a series of 36 bone lesions in the mandible and the maxilla were described in patients undergoing treatment with pamidronate or zoledronate [12].

Then in 2007, the American Association of Oral and Maxillofacial Surgeons (AAOMS) described osteonecrosis of the jaws like persistent bone exposure in the mouth for over 8 weeks in patients with a history of use of bisphosphonates, without local evidence of malignancy or radiotherapeutic treatment of the affected region [15].

Despite that the term osteonecrosis has been used in numerous contexts and even in different locations (not only for the jaws); it is currently related exclusively to the chronic use of bisphosphonates. The condition is called bisphosphonate-related osteonecrosis of the jaw (BRONJ) [16], which was changed by the AAOMS in 2014 for the term medication-related osteonecrosis of the jaw (MRONJ), since this complication has also been described in relation to other antiresorptive drugs (denosumab) and antiagiogenic therapies [17].

1.2.1. Prevalence and incidence

The prevalence of osteonecrosis of the jaws is variable according to the consulted authors, reaching approximately 7–12%, although in more recent articles it tends to be even higher (18.6%) [18].

In regards to IV bisphosphonates, the bibliography of a series of cases, case studies and controls and cohorts, the estimations of the accumulated incidence of MRONJ ranges from 0.8 to 12% [19].

In regards to oral bisphosphonates, clinical effectiveness has been proven, which is shown in over 190 million prescriptions of these drugs around the globe [20]. Despite that osteonecrosis cases have been described, these patients have a considerably lower risk of MRONJ than cancer patients who have been treated with monthly IV bisphosphonates.

According to the database of the alendronate manufacturer (Merk), the incidence of MRONJ was calculated as 0.7/100.000 people/years of exposure [21]. This derives from the number of (non-confirmed) reports of the cases that were considered as MRONJ, divided between the number of alendronate pills prescribed since the approval of the drug. Although this is the best information available to date, there could be a bias in the collection and validity of the data.

In Australia, MRONJ incidence in patients receiving weekly alendronate treatment ranges between 0.01 and 0.04% [22]

Felsenberg registered a prevalence of MRONJ among patients who underwent bisphosphonates therapy for osteoporosis of 0.00038%, based on the reports of three cases in the German Central Register for Jaw Necrosis [23].

1.3. Risk factors

1.3.1. Local factors

A. Dentoalveolar surgery

- Extractions

- Dental implants
- Periapical surgery
- Periodontal surgery

Cancer patients treated with IV bisphosphonates and who underwent dentoalveolar procedures had 5–21 times more risk of MRONJ than cancer patients who were treated with IV bisphosphonates and who did not undergo dentoalveolar procedures [19].

B. Local anatomy

B1. *Mandibular*

- Lingual torus
- Mylohyoid line

B2. *Maxilla*

- Palatine Torus

The lesions are located with a higher frequency on the mandible than on the superior maxilla (2:1) and more frequently in areas with thin mucosa that cover bone protrusions, such as the torus, bone exostosis and the mylohyoid edge [24–26].

C. Concomitant oral diseases: Dental or periodontal abscesses [27].

1.3.2. Systemic and demographic factors

a. Age: Advanced age is related to a higher prevalence of MRONJ.

b. Sex: This factor has not been statistically related to a higher risk of osteonecrosis.

c. Race: Caucasians have a higher risk of MRONJ compared to the Negro race [28].

d. Cancer diagnosis, with or without osteoporosis: The type of malignancy is not statistically related to a higher risk of MRONJ, although the presence of bone metastasis presents a correlation, according to Wessel's article (P = 0.051) [29]. It is related with a higher risk of osteonecrosis in the coadjuvant treatments in these patients, such as chemotherapeutic agents (cyclophosphamide), erythropoietin and steroids [30, 31].

e. Tobacco and alcohol: There is a possible correlation with smoking but not with drinking, according to the study published by Wessel et al. [29].

f. Genetic factors: It has been proven that polymorphism in the farnesyl pyrophosphate synthase or the cytochrome of gen P450 CYP2C8 increase the risk of MRONJ in patients treated with IV bisphosphonates [32–34].

g. Others: Dialysis, low hemoglobin, obesity and diabetes are variables related to MRONJ [29, 31, 35].

1.3.3. Drug-related factors

a. **Bisphosphonate potency**: IV bisphosphonates present higher power than oral ones [19].

b. **Duration of the treatment**: The longer the duration of the treatment, higher the risk of MRONJ [19].

1.4. Diagnosis

Patients diagnosed with MRONJ are defined by the following characteristics [17]:

1. Prior treatment with antiresorptive and antiangiogenic drugs.
2. Presence of bone exposure or intra- or extraoral fistula for over 8 weeks, without remission.
3. Patients who have not been treated with radiotherapy nor have metastasizing diseases in the jaws.

With the intention of standardizing all the signs and symptoms present in the patients affected by osteonecrosis of the jaws, a protocol for MRONJ diagnosis was proposed in 2010 [36].

1.4.1. Clinical diagnosis

a. **Greater clinical signs** [37]

- Exposed necrotic bone in the oral cavity

b. **Minor clinical signs and symptoms**

- Abscess
- Displacement of jaw fragments
- Intra-extra oral fistula
- Jaw deformation
- Lip hypaesthesia/paraesthesia
- Gum or mucous fistula
- Nasal level excretions
- Unhealed post-extraction alveoli
- Pus excretion
- Spontaneous expulsion of bone sequestration

- Dental mobility
- Local inflammation
- Bone and dental pain
- Trismus

1.4.2. Radiographic/tomographic diagnosis

a. **Initial signs** [38]

- Cortical fracture
- Sclerosis of the focal bone marrow
- Presence of post-extraction alveoli
- Trabecular engrossment

b. **Late signs**

- Diffuse sclerosis
- Oro-antral fistula
- Osteolysis extended to the sinus floor
- Osteosclerosis of adjacent bones (zygoma and hard palate)
- Pathological fracture
- Prominence of the lower dental nerve canal
- Sinusitis

1.4.3. Diagnosis through complementary testing

The histopathologic study and microbiological culture are also tests developed on the suppuration area. Developing an antibiogram is very helpful since these patients will be treated with antibiotics during long periods of time and it is convenient to know the existing bacterial spectrum and the sensitivity of these microorganisms to different antibiotics.

1.5. MRONJ staging

The stages initially described by Ruggiero et al. [24] have been modified and adapted to classify patients with greater precision [17, 19, 39] (**Figure 1**).

Risk patient: Without apparent necrotic lesions in asymptomatic patients undergoing treatments with oral or IV bisphosphonates.

http://dx.doi.org/10.5772/intechopen.69315

Stage 0: Patients without clinical evidence of bone necrosis, but with unspecific systems or clinical or radiographic findings.

a. **Symptoms**

- Odontalgia without odontogenic cause.
- Pain at the jaw level that may irradiate to the temporomandibular joint.
- Sinus pain, which may be related to inflammation or engrossment of the maxillary sinus wall.
- Alteration of the neurosensory function

b. **Clinical findings**

- Dental loss without periodontal cause
- Periapical or periodontal fistula that is not related to a pulpal necrosis by cavities.

c. **Radiographic findings**

- Bone resorption that is not attributable to chronic periodontal disease.
- Changes to the trabeculate and bone density and resistance to healing of the post-extraction alveoli.
- Widening/darkening of the periodontal ligament.
- Narrowing of the lower dental nerve canal.

These unspecific findings that are characteristic of State 0 can take place in patients with a prior history of more advanced phases in whom the disease has been cured and have no clinical evidence of exposed bone.

Stage 1: Asymptomatic bone exposure without clinical signs of inflammation or infection.

Stage 2: Bone exposure with infection and pain, erythema or inflammation of the mucosa, with our without suppuration.

Stage 3: Bone exposure associated to pain, inflammation and infection with one or more of the following complications:

- Exposed necrotic bone beyond the alveolar region, as the lower border of the mandibular branch, maxillary sinus or zygoma.
- Pathological fracture.
- Oro-antral and oro-nasal communication.
- Extra-oral fistula.

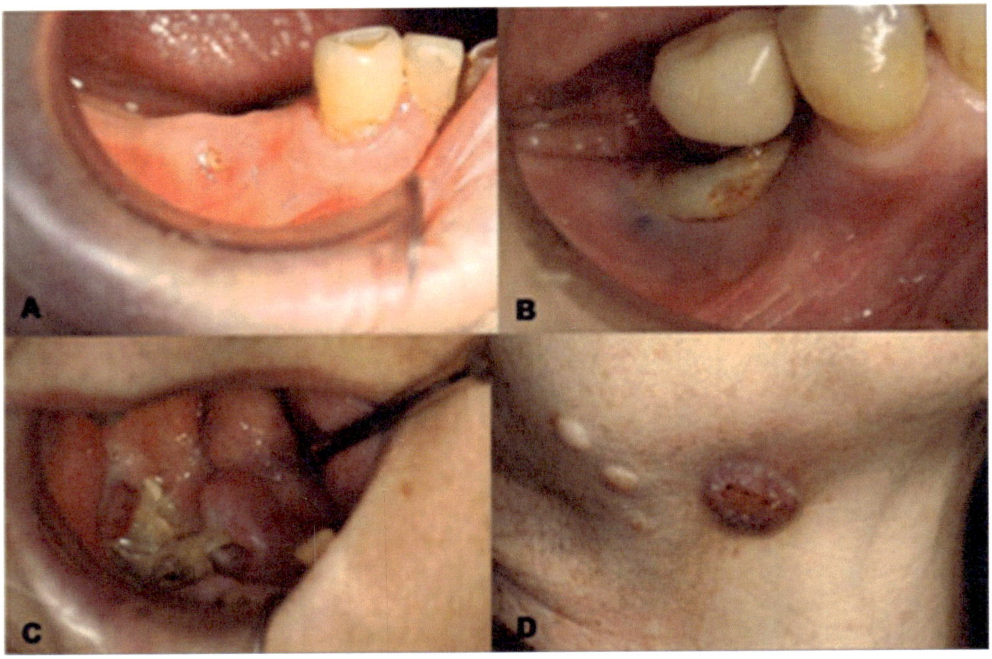

Figure 1. TNM Staging. (A) Stage 1; (B) Stage 2; (C) and (D) Stage 3.

1.6. Treatment

To focus on the treatment to be developed regarding this complication, it is essential to know the pathophysiology of MRONJ, only by this way we can draft an appropriate treatment plan.

To date, the source has not been adequately documented, describing a multi factor source. Suppression of bone remodeling can contribute to the development of osteonecrosis by an inadequate activity of osteoclasts that do not allow the post-extraction alveoli to heal. The presence of microflora in the mouth have also been related as an osteonecrosis-promoting factor, since numerous biopsy studies and bone sequestrations revealed the presence of *Fusobacterium, Eikenella, Bacillus, Actinomyces, Staphylococcus* and *Streptococcus* [40]. Bacterial infection produces local cytokines that promote local osteolysis that contribute to the stimulation of bone resorption and, therefore, subsequent necrosis [41–43].

Additionally, recent articles relate the presence of Actinomyces in MRONJ, although these are small studies on a series of cases having a very small impact in establishing a specific treatment strategy [28, 44–46].

Antinomyces are Gram-positive anaerobic facultative bacteria that do not form spores and are commonly filamentous. They are frequent commensals of the mucosa in the oropharynx, intestinal tract and the female genital tract, once the mucosa barrier is broken due to trauma, surgical interventions or foreign objects, they can invade deep tissue structures and compromise treatment response. Progressive chronic disease is called actinomycosis, and the treatment of this pathology is based on a prolonged antimicrobial therapy for 2–6 months in combination with surgery [47, 48].

1.6.1. Conservative treatment

a. **Oral hygiene**: Teach the patient good brushing techniques and a good daily control of dental plaque.

b. **Periodical dental exam**: Periodical visits to control the new pathology that could receive conservative treatment.

c. **Antimicrobial rinses**: The mouthwash par excellence is chlorhexidine at 0.12%.

d. **Antibiotic treatment**: Multiple antibiotic standards have been described, but it is obvious that there is an increasing bacterial resistance to penicillins. Running an antibiogram is always advisable to assess the sensitivity and drug resistance to provide the most appropriate treatment.

- Amoxicillin with or without clavulanic acid (500 mg/l g)
- Clindamycin (300 mg)
- Azithromycin (500 mg)
- Metronidazole with betalactamic antibiotics

e. **Ozone therapy**: Ozone is a natural gas produced by the atmosphere that has antimicrobial and healing properties. Its role as a treatment for the osteonecrosis of the jaws has been discussed in clinical and pre-clinical studies, since it was believe that this gas induced tissue repair and, therefore, healing of the mucosa [49].

Numerous studies have used this therapy as an adjuvant in antibiotic treatments with good results, although further standardized studies are needed to accurately determine their effectiveness [50].

f. **Hyperbaric oxygen therapy**: Hyperbaric oxygen therapy (HBOT) is very controversial in the literature. It is believed that it stimulates tissue healing, reducing edema and inflammation, stimulates cell proliferation and moderates the suppression of bone remodeling produced by the use of bisphosphonates [51–53].

g. **Soft LASER**: This innovative and effective medical method has a pain-reducing effect, improving circulation in the lesion and helping nerve regeneration. At an oral level, it improves re-epithelialization following periodontal or third molar surgery [52, 54].

Most conservative treatments on their own do not show accurate results on their effectiveness, especially in more advance stages. Authors use them in combination with antibiotics and observe that these can help heal the patient, especially in terms of tissue regeneration; but it is always reinforced with an appropriate antibiotic treatment (**Table 1**) [55].

1.6.2. Surgical treatment

For patients in advanced stages and resistant-clinical-cases:

a. Conservative surgery: Includes the remotion of the necrotic bone (sequestration) and/or superficial unbinding associated to antibiotic therapy and chlorhexidine rinses.

b. Resective surgery: Destined to patients in whom previous treatments have not been effective or have very advanced stages. This process has been questioned since it is difficult to guarantee complete resection of the necrosed bone sectioned at the healthy bone [56, 57].

Numerous studies show high improvement rates in patients who underwent surgical treatment both in conservative and resective procedures (**Table 2**) [55].

1.6.3. Other treatments

The use of stem cells [58, 59], platelet-rich plasma [60], the administration of parathyroid hormone [61] or the use of leukocyte- and platelet-rich fibrin [62] are also promising proposals, but they require further clinical studies that attest to their effectiveness.

1.6.4. Protocol for the treatment of MRONJ

Risk Patients: They do not require treatment, but must be informed of the risks of developing MRONJ, as well as the signs and symptoms of this disease [19, 24].

Type of treatment	Author/Year	No. patients healed/No. patients treated (%)
Antibiotic treatment	Melea et al. (2014)	23/38 (60%)
	Van den Wyngaert et al. (2009)	16/33 (53%)
	Scoletta et al. (2010)	18/30 (62%)
	Nicolatou-Galitis et al. (2011)	7/47 (14.9%)
T Antibiotic treatment + hyperbaric oxygen	Freiberger et al. (2012)	13/25 (52%)
Antibiotic treatment + ozone therapy	Ripamonti et al. (2011)	10/10 (100%)
Pentoxifylline + α-tocopherol	Magremanne et al. (2014)	1/1 (100%)

Table 1. Summary of studies with a conservative focus for the management of ONJ-related osteonecrosis [55].

Type of treatment	Author/Year	No. patients healed/No. patients treated (%)
Conservative surgery	Rugani et al. 2014	15/17 (88.2%)
	Vescovi et al. (2012)	11/17 (65%)
	Thumbigere-Math et al. (2009)	3/19 (15%)
	Williamson et al. (2010)	40/40 (100%)
	Vescovi et al. (2014)	25/27 (92.6%)
	Graziani et al. (2012)	227 (54%)
	Wutzl et al. (2008)	24/41 (519%)
Conservative surgery + ozone therapy	Agrillo et al.	57/94 (60%)
Conservative surgery + L-PRF	Kim et al.	26/34 (77%)
Resect1ve surgery	Graziani et al. (2012)	87/120 (72.5%)
	Carlson and Basile (2009)	87/95 (92%)
	Bedogni et al. (2011)	27/30 (90%)
	Voss et al. (2012)	20/21 (95%)
	Schubert et al. (2012)	47/54 (87%)

Note: L-PRF (leukocyte- and platelet-rich fibrin).

Table 2. Summary of studies with a surgical focus for the treatment of MRONJ.

Stage 0: Symptomatic treatment and control of local factors, such as cavities and periodontal disease.

Stage 1: Daily rinses with antimicrobial agents (chlorhexidine at 0.12%) and regular control visits.

Stage 2: Oral antimicrobial rinses (chlorhexidine at 0.12%) in combination with antibiotic therapy.

Stage 3: Combination of different protocols:

- Surgical debridement of the necrotic bone
- Antibiotic therapy (oral or IV)
- Analgesics
- Daily rinses with antimicrobial agents (chlorhexidine at 0.12%)

Regardless of the state of the patient, mobile bone sequestration segments must be retrieved. Extraction of affected teeth with symptoms within the exposed necrotic bone must be considered, since it is improbable that the extraction exacerbates the established necrotic process.

1.7. Prevention

Despite all the treatments proposed above, the latest articles agree that none of these are completely effective for all cases, therefore, the main goal in these patients is prevention of this complication.

Back in 2009, AAOMS [16] determined that prevention was the main goal in the management of these patients, recommending that patients are evaluated and treated before initiating bisphosphonate therapy.

There are several studies that document that preventative dental treatment decreases the risk of MRONJ among patients with malignant tumors treated with IV bisphosphonates [63, 64]. These findings suggest that, although MRONJ is not eliminated, evaluations and dental treatment prior to beginning bisphosphonate therapy in cancer patients reduces the risk of MRONJ.

Furthermore, they advise revising the doses prescribed to the patients, since it has been proven that [65] the accumulative doses can increase the risk of suffering complications.

The risk of developing MRONJ due to oral bisphosphonate treatment is minimal, but it seems to increase when the duration of the treatment is more than 3 years. This period of time can be reduced in the presence of certain concomitant diseases, such as the chronic use of corticosteroids. Systemic conditions permitting the clinician should consider interrupting oral bisphosphonate treatments for a 3-month period before and another 3 months after elective invasive dental surgery with the purpose of reducing the risk of MRONJ. The justification of this focus is based on extrapolated data that show fluctuations depending on osteoclasts, which is related to the treatment with bisphosphonates, and recent studies show that there is a better result in the treatment of MRONJ after eliminating the drug [66]. In the long term, prospective studies will be necessary to establish the efficacy of suppression period of these drugs to reduce the risk of MRONJ in patients undergoing oral bisphosphonate treatments.

1.7.1. Patients about to begin bisphosphonate treatment

The goal is to reduce the risk of developing MRONJ to the minimum despite that a small percentage of patients who receive IV bisphosphonate therapy can develop osteonecrosis spontaneously [19]. Thus, if the medical conditions of the patient allow, the start of the treatment must be delayed until their dental health is optimal [63, 64]. This decision must be made by the doctor, together with the dentist and other specialists involved in the patient's care.

Untreatable teeth and those with bad prognosis must be extracted. Additionally, other necessary dentoalveolar surgeries should also be performed at this time. The start of the treatment with bisphosphonates, if possible, should be delayed until complete healing of the mucosa (14–21 days) or until there is an appropriate bone healing.

Dental prophylaxis, cavity control and restorative-conservative odontology are essential to maintain dental health. This level of attention should be maintained indefinitely. The patients with complete or partial prosthesis should be examined to avoid the trauma areas of the mucosa, especially in the border of the tongue. It is essential that patients are trained in regards to the importance of oral hygiene and regular dental evaluations, and instructed specifically to report any pain, swelling or exposed bone area.

1.7.2. Asymptomatic patients who receive IV bisphosphonates

Procedures that imply direct bone lesion should be avoided, therefore, unrestorable teeth should be treated by eliminating the crown and the endodontic treatment of root fragments [21]. The placement of dental implants must be avoided in cancer patients exposed to higher potency bisphosphonates (zoledronic acid and pamidronate) with a frequent dose program (4–12 times/year).

1.7.3. Asymptomatic patients who receive oral bisphosphonate treatments

In general terms, these patients seem to have less severe manifestations of necrosis and respond promptly to the described treatments [67, 68]. Elective alveolodental surgery does not seem to be contraindicated in this group, although it is advisable that the patients are appropriately informed on the small risk of complications in bone healing. The use of levels in the bone exchange markers and a drug break in the treatment have been documented as additional tools that guide in making treatment decisions in patients exposed to oral bisphosphonates [68]. Currently, the effectiveness of the systemic markers of bone exchange to assess the risk of developing jaw necrosis in risk patients is being questioned, which requires more research before considering it as a valid risk evaluation tool. In the long term, prospective studies will be necessary to establish the efficacy of suppression period of these drugs (drug holidays) to reduce the risk of MRONJ in these patients.

The risk of MRONJ seems to be more associated to the duration of the treatment (≥3 years) than the dosage, since there has not been any information indicating that the monthly dosage of bisphosphonates is related, with a high or reduced risk of MRONJ when it is compared with the weekly dose program.

There a no solid recommendations based on clinical research for patients who take oral bisphosphonates. The Task Force strategies described above have remained essentially unchanged and are based on the clinical experience of the physicians (expert opinions) who participate in the care of these patients [24, 64, 68–70].

1.7.3.1. Patients who have taken oral bisphosphonates for less than 3 years and have no clinical risk factors, alterations and have the possibility of programmed surgery

Includes all the common procedures for oral and maxillofacial surgeons, periodontists and specialists.

If dental implants are placed, an informed consent must be presented in regards to possible implant failure and the possible osteonecrosis of the jaws, if the patient continues the oral bisphosphonate treatment. It is also advisable to contact the doctor who initially prescribed the oral bisphosphonate to suggest monitoring of these patients and consider a possible alternative dose to the bisphosphonate, temporary suppression of the drug or an alternative to the medication.

1.7.3.2. Patients who have been administered oral bisphosphonates for less than 3 years associated with corticosteroids

If systemic conditions allow, the physician must be contacted to consider the interruption of the oral treatment for at least 3 months prior to the oral surgery. Reinstatement of bisphosphonate therapy should not take place until complete bone healing. These strategies are based on the opinion of experts with significant clinical experience and the hypothesis that concomitant treatment with corticosteroids can increase the risk of developing MRONJ.

1.7.3.3. Patients who have been administered oral bisphosphonates for less than 3 years, with or without corticosteroids

If systemic conditions allow, the physician must be contacted to consider the interruption of the oral treatment for at least 3 months prior to the oral surgery and, similarly, bisphosphonate therapy should not be reinstated until complete bone healing.

1.7.4. CTXs (C-terminal telopeptide in serum)

This bone resorption biomarker has been used for years as a predictive factor for the development of bisphosphonate-related osteonecrosis when deciding on the dental treatments for this type of patients [71]. In a study by Marx et al. (2007), they observed CTXs in fasting samples to correlate the values and the period of use of oral bisphosphonates and to demonstrate if the increase in value could indicate a recovery in bone remodeling when suspending oral bisphosphonate treatment. Risk stratification was determined according to the obtained values, CTX under 100 pg/ml represented high risk, CTX between 100 pg/ml and 150 pg/ml represented moderate risk, while CTX above 150 pg/ml represented minimal risk. CTX values increased between 25.9 and 26.4 pg/ml for each drug holiday month from the bisphosphonates, which indicated a recovery of the bone remodeling and a directive in terms of when the oral surgical procedures could be developed at a lower risk. Additionally, it was observed that in terms of the drug suppression periods associated to CTX values, the latter rose above the threshold of 150 pg/ml, which coincides with spontaneous bone healing or a better response to complete healing after debridement. [68].

After years of research, a meta-analysis of nine controlled studies did not reveal significant differences in the mean values of CTXs among patients with MRONJ and controls (mean difference, −31.417; 95% confidence interval [CI], −91.560 to 28.726; P = 0.306). Additionally, a second meta-analysis of four studies did not show significant differences in the risk of osteonecrosis with CTX values below 150 pg/ml for patients with MRONJ in comparison with the controls (risk ratio, 1.892; 95% CI, 0.636–5.626; P = 0.251) [71].

http://dx.doi.org/10.5772/intechopen.69315

The term **"Drug Holiday"** has appeared recently as a preventative measure when certain risk odontological treatment must be performed or to improve healing after the appearance of osteonecrosis. There are several proposals but there is no clear consensus regarding bisphosphonate suppression periods (**Table 3**) [72].

Cancer patients benefit mainly from the therapeutic effects of bisphosphonates, such as the control of bone pain and the incidence of pathological fractures. An interruption of IV bisphosphonate therapy does not offer short-term benefits. However, if systemic conditions allow, long-term suspension can be beneficial in the stabilization of the areas affected by MRONJ, which reduces the risk of necrosis in other locations and minimizes clinical symptoms [63, 64]. The oncologist's role is very important to assess the risks and benefits of suppressing the treatment.

Regarding the interruption of oral bisphosphonate treatment in patients with MRONJ, a gradual improvement of the disease has been proven [68]. The interruption of oral bisphosphonates for 6–12 months may favor healing, after the removal of a bone sequestration or after

Guideline	Bisphosphonate exposure history by route of administration	
	Oral	**Intravenous**
ASBMR[56]	No specific guidelines given	No guidelines given
AAOMS[57]	Less than 3 year duration:	No guidelines given
	No change to dosing	
	Less than 3 year duration and corticosteroids:	
	Cease: 3 months prior	
	Recommence: Osseous healing has occurred†	
	More than 3 year duration:	
	Cease: 3 months prior	
	Recommence: Osseous healing has occurred†	
CCPG[60]	No specific guidelines given	Cease: 3–6 months prior
		Recommence: Full healing†
Mayo Clinic[62]	No guidelines given	Cease: 1 month prior
		Recommence: Full healing
MFA[64]	No guidelines given	Low/intermediate risk of SRE:
		Cease: 2–3 months prior
		Recommence: 2–3 months after or full healing

†If systemic condition permits.

Table 3. Proposals in the bisphosphonates suppression rate [72].

debridement. The decision to suppress the drug must be assessed by the physician and the patient, as long as the systemic conditions allow.

2. Bisphosphonates

2.1. Definition

Bisphosphonates are non-metabolizable pyrophosphate analogues that are deposited on the bones and prevent or improve bone complications of the patients with bone alterations. Different bisphosphonates differ depending on the alterations of the R-2 lateral chain structure. These R-2 lateral chains determine the efficiency and the cellular effects of the inhibition of bone resorption [73]. The bisphosphonates are internalized by osteoclasts, causing the interruption of bone resorption. They also have antigiogenic properties, since they reduce the circulating levels of vascular endothelial growth factor (VEGF) [74–78] and antineoplastic effects [79]. It has very little intestinal absorption and is excreted without being metabolized by the kidneys.

Until 2001, pamidronate (Aredia®) was the only drug approved in the USA for the treatment of bone metastasis. In 2002, the US Food and Drug Administration (FDA) [80] approved zoledronic acid (Zometa®) as a treatment for these patients. Currently, the annual transfusion of zoledronate (Reclast®) and the parenteral formulation of ibandronate (Bonviva®) administered every 3 months has been approved by the FDA for the treatment of osteoporosis [81].

In 2003, using the articles by Marx [12] and Ruggiero et al. [25], they observed and reported on the cases of unhealed bone exposure in the maxillofacial region in patients treated with IV bisphosphonates and, after multiple further publications, in September 2004, Novartis the manufacturer of pamidronate (Aredia®) and zoledronic acid (Zometa), added the complications deriving from this treatment to the labeling of these drugs, with the purpose of warning the health care professionals of the possibility of developing osteonecrosis of the jaws [82].

2.2. Types of bisphosphonates

According to their chemical structure, these are divided into two groups.

Non-nitrogenous: These are very similar to natural pyrophosphate, such as etidronate or clodronate that contain CH3 and Cl groups instead of the R2 chain and a nitrogen-free ring, such as tiludronate. They are metabolized by macrophages in toxic analogues of adenosine triphosphate (ATP) [83].

Nitrogenous: They present higher power, such as zoledronate and pamidronate, with a primary atom of basic nitrogen with an alkyl chain. They have a power 10–100 times higher than non-nitrogenous. Mevalonate inhibits the cholesterol route through the farnesyl diphosphate synthase enzyme [83].

There is a great variety of bisphosphonates approved for clinical use in the USA (**Table 4**).

Generic name	Commercial name	Laboratory	RP	FDA-a
Pamidronate	Aredia, IV	Novartis	100	1991
Tiludronate	Skelid, O	Sanofi	10	1997
Alendronate	Fosamax, O	Merck	1000	1997
Etidronate	Didronel, O	Proctor & Gamble	1	1997
Risedronate	Actonel, O	Proctor & Gamble	5000	1998
Zoledrónic acid	Zometa, IV	Novartis	100,000	2001
Ibandronate	Bonviva, O	Roche	10,000	2005

Note: O: oral; IV: intravenous.

Table 4. Drugs approved in EEUU.

2.2.1. *IV bisphosphonates*

It is estimated that over 2.8 million cancer patients from around the world have received treatment with IV bisphosphonates since their introduction [84].

- **Pamidronate** (Aredia): a second-generation bisphosphonates that are administered every 3–4 weeks at a dosage of 90 mg.
- **Zoledronic acid** (Zometa): a third-generation bisphosphonates, administered every 3–4 weeks, at a dosage of 4 mg.

It is a heterocyclic imidazole and, to date, the most powerful bisphosphonate to be administered to humans. In a test on in-vitro bone resorption using mouse cranium, zoledronate was at least 100 times more powerful than pamidronate. Additionally, the in-vivo animal model of calcitriol-induced hypercalcemia in thyroparathyroidectomized rats was 850 times more active than pamidronate and over 4 times more powerful than clodronate. Of all the bisphosphonates under clinical evaluation, this is the one having a higher therapeutic relationship between the desired inhibition of bone resorption and the undesired inhibition of bone mineralization, furthermore, several toxicology studies proved that the compound is safe [85].

2.2.2. *Oral bisphosphonates*

Due to the proven clinical effectiveness, it is considered a first line therapy in the treatment of osteoporosis and they are the most prescribed antiresorptive agents.

- **Alendronate** (Fosamax): 70 mg once a week during the osteoporosis treatment or less, if it has been prescribed for the prevention of osteoporosis.

It has been proven to prevent approximately 50% of cases in the prevention of the bone loss in the spine or hips in menopausal women and the reduction of bone fractures [86, 87].

- **Risedronate** (Actonel): 35 mg once a week.

In a prospective study with a large sample, risedronate produced a reduction of 30% in hip fractures [88, 89].

- **Ibandronate** (Boniva): is the latest drug to be approved by the FDA (March, 2005) for the treatment of osteoporosis and it is administered monthly.
- **Etidronate** (Didronel): prescribed for the Paget disease with a dose of 300–750 mg/day for 6 months.
- **Tiludronate** (Skelid): prescribed for Paget disease with a dose of 400 mg/day for 3 months.

2.3. Metabolism

Bisphosphonates have an average life between 30 min and 2 h and are deposited in the locations with higher bone metabolism, and can remain at the bone level for approximately 10 years. The highest concentration is located in urine and saliva, and the most frequent adverse effects are renal insufficiency and osteonecrosis [90–92]. The accumulative doses described by Maerevoet, is of 72 mg for 18 months [90, 93].

In the case of IV bisphosphonates, such as zolendronic acid, 40% is eliminated unaltered through urine after 24 h [94] and the remaining 60% are united at bone level due to the great affinity of hydroxyapatite. This phenomenon takes place in areas of bone remodeling, in which the periodical exchange produces unaltered kidney excretion after a long elimination phase [95]. The mean life of this second elimination phase may last months or years, depending on the duration of the bisphosphonate treatment [96].

Excretion of oral bisphosphonates has also been studied, for example, in a rat study, in which they administered risedronate orally, and determined that 80% of the drug was excreted through the kidneys 12 h after the administration of the drug. Additionally, the study concluded that taking oral bisphosphonates with mineral water that contains high calcium and magnesium levels reduced the effect of the drug; therefore it is advisable to take it as soon as the patient wakes up and in a vertical position [97]. These authors previously described the effect of water in combination with taking alendronate [98].

2.4. Detection of bisphosphonates

The concentration of bisphosphonates in a specific bone location depends on the speed of bone remodeling and blood circulation [99]. It is important to know the concentration of accumulated bisphosphonate in the bone to understand the long-term drug effect and its toxicity. Today, numerous authors have been able to quantify these drugs in plasma and urine through mass spectrometry (MS), which requires a previous derivation process that allows to transform the bisphosphonates into more hydrophobic substances so they can be studied [100, 101].

The development of analysis methods for the detection of bisphosphonates in biological matrices, it is hard due to the chemical properties of these compounds. The detection of bisphosphonates in human biological matrices comes with certain difficulties and therefore a broad range of analytic techniques have been described, such as gas chromatography [102], ion chromatography [103], capillary electrophoresis, ionization mass spectrometry by electrospray [104] and chromatography of fluids [105].

2.4.1. *Mass spectrometry (MS)*

A method for the extraction and detection of zoledronic acid in urine and blood plasma or even accumulated in the bone (in a mouse model) through the combination of chromatography and mass spectrometry (MS) [100, 106].

In these studies, a higher accumulation of bisphosphonates in bone extracts of the mandible was detected, compared to other types of bones [106]. On the other hand, human urine and blood plasma detected a maximum concentration peak of the drug of 77 μM (5 h after the administration) and 1.5 μM (after 1 h), respectively [100]. This methodology achieves high sensitivity and specificity in the detection, however, it requires a pretty complex and arduous treatment of the sample requiring phases with chemical reactions to derive the complex. The complexity of the treatment of the sample can be a limiting factor when the number of samples to be analyzed is high, as in the case of the follow-up of the pharmacokinetics and the bioavailability of zoledronic acid since its administration. For this reason, it would be desirable to have a more efficient alternative method to detect this drug.

2.4.2. *Nuclear magnetic resonance spectroscopy (NMR)*

Nuclear magnetic resonance (NMR) spectroscopy is a useful technique in chemometrics that can be used for the characterization of simple or complex mixes of different sources and provide quantitative results. There is a great variety of "omics" applications for NMR, such as *metabonomics, metabolomics, proteomics, transcriptomics, fluxomics, foodomics, lipidomics, fermentanomics, isotopomics,* etc. One of the areas with greater impact in biomedicine is metabolomics by NMR for the study of metabolites in different types of samples, such as biofluids (urine, saliva, blood plasma, blood serum, sweat, etc.), tissue extracts, cerebrospinal fluid, cells, etc. Metabolomics by NMR can be used to find biomarkers for the study, diagnosis and prognosis of diseases. Similarly, it can help many traditional analysis at a clinical level, since the cost per sample is or can be competitive if large lots of samples are managed, in terms of the time for the analysis (measurement) and the generation of results (automated). There are a number of pathologies for which the study of biofluids or tissues by NMR has found useful biomarkers [107, 108]. A relevant case of application of NMR in this area is the quantification of lipoprotein in blood serum/plasma. NMR offers details on the relative abundance of different subclasses of lipoproteins that are not accessible to traditional analysis methods [109, 110].

It is a quantitative technique that allows determination of the absolute concentration of diluted substances in general, including biofluids. It is based on the fact that the intensity of a signal in the NMR spectrum is proportionate to the concentration of the molecule (or metabolite) generating the said signal. As an approximate value, to assess the sensitivity of this technique, in a current spectrometer with a 11.7 T magnet, the minimum concentration required to detect a molecule in a monodimensional spectrum (1D) of ^{1}H (proton spectrum, as it is commonly known in our jargon) must amount to a minimum of 10 μm, for a measurement period of 15 min.

For the case of urine samples, under these same measurement conditions, 50–60 metabolites can be identified and quantified in their proton spectrum (**Figure 2**).

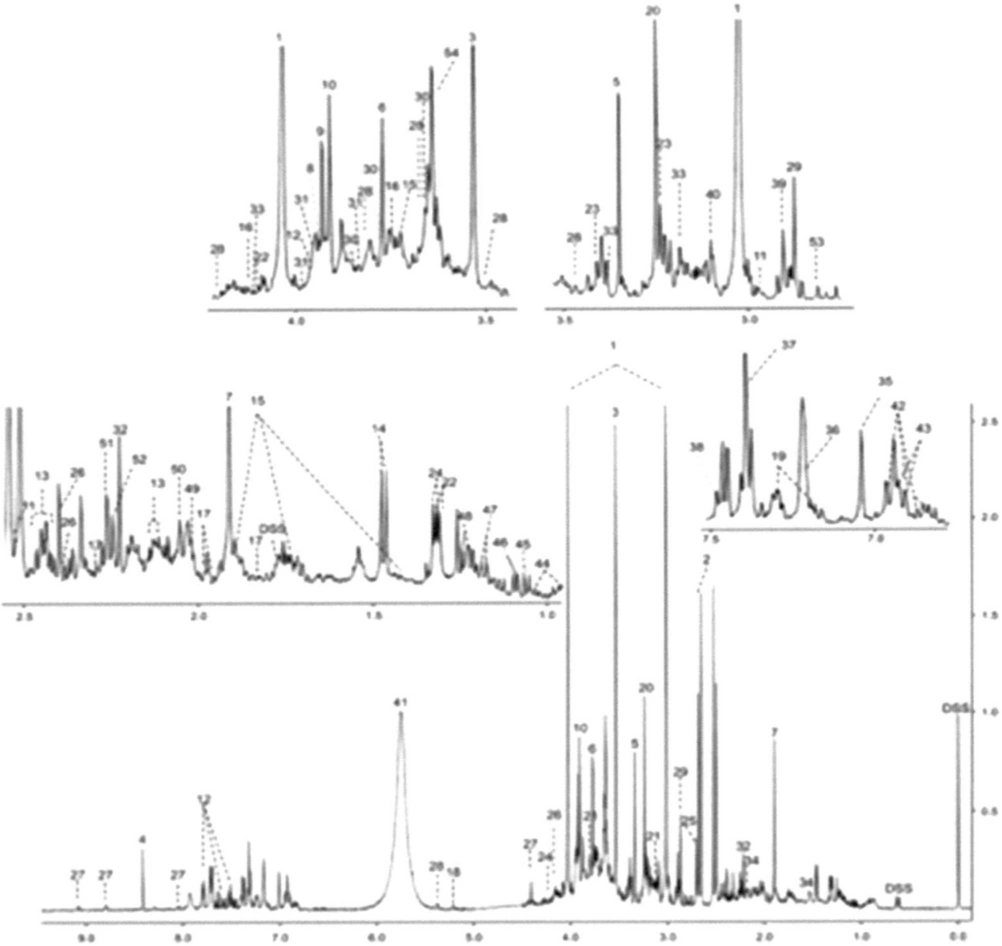

Figure 2. Typical spectrum of ^{1}H NMR of a human urine sample. The numbers indicate the following metabolites: 1: creatinine, 2: citric acid, 3: glycine, 4: formic acid, 5: methanol, 6: guanidinoacetic acid, 7: acetic acid, 8: L-cysteine, 9: glycolic acid, 10: creatine, 11: Isocitric acid, 12: hippuric acid, 13: L-glutamine, 14: L-alanine, 15: L-Lysine, 16: gluconic acid, 17: 2-hidoxiglutaric acid, 18: D-glucose, 19: indoxyl sulfate, 20: trimethyl-N-oxide, 21: ethanolamine, 22: L-lactic acid, 23: taurine, 24: L-threonine, 25: dimethylamine, 26: pyroglutamic acid, 27: trigonelline, 28: sucrose, 29: trimethylamine, 30: mannitol, 31: L-serine, 32: acetone, 33: L-cystine, 34: adipic acid, 35: L-histidine, 36: L-tyrosine, 37: imidazole, 38: mandelic acid, 39: dimethylglycine, 40: cis-aconitic acid, 41: urea, 42: 3-(3-Hydroxyphenyl)-3-hydroxypropanoic (HPHPA), 43: phenol, 45: isobutyric acid, 46: methylsuccinic acid, 47: 3-Aminoisobutíric acid, 48: L-fucose, 49: N-acetylaspartic acid, 50: N-acetylneuraminic, 51: acetoacetic acid, 52: Alpha-aminoadipic acid, 53: methylguanidine, 54: phenylacetylglutamine [111].

When a series of NMR spectra need to be compared, such as urine, it is important to consider some details regarding post-processing of the spectra and the process to obtain their quantitative values, in such a way that no errors are introduced in this phase and the quantitative results that are obtained are the most precise and repeatable as possible. Although with slight variations regarding some details, the general method for the treatment of spectral information for the metabolomic studies by NMR is the one described below.

2.4.2.1. Preparation of a biofluid sample

A series of protocols have been established for the preparation of biofluid samples and their subsequent preservation until the NMR measuring [112, 113]. Similarly, there are experimental parameters to be used for the measurement of the NMR spectrum for each type of biofluid [112, 113]. These protocols standardize the measurements, thus allowing the comparison of the spectra obtained and the NMR spectrum (e.g. the Human Metabolome Database: www.hmdb.ca) and/or with bibliographic results. These sample preparation protocols tend to be simple and do not require special laboratory equipment.

2.4.2.1.1. Generation of a signal intensity data matrix (integrals) on regions of interest (ROIs) of the NMR spectrum

The raw data provided by the spectrometer when measuring the ^{1}H NMR spectrum is called free induction decay (FID). The data must be post-processed by applying a series of operations to generate a final spectrum with a scale of frequencies (expressed by standardized ppm units) and with the best quality possible [114]. Once the post-processing has been completed for each of the spectra to be studied, the following phase consists of comparing analogue regions of the spectrum with the target to find, if possible, a certain region that could serve as a biomarker, in other words, a region in which the signal's intensity pattern is significantly different in the samples of the control group and the experiment group, while being similar within their own group.

Instead of manually selecting one or several regions for comparison, the usual and practical procedure is to perform a systematic analysis, dividing the entire spectrum automatically, from right to left, through a series of small segmental regions (e.g. with an established width) in which the area of the signal is integrated individually. Each of these regions is called buckets or regions of interest (ROIs). This way, a complete spectrum is represented as a data vector formed by the integrals of the selected ROIs, with as many integral values as segments of the spectrum have been created.

Lastly, a table is created with the data, placing the vectors of each of the analyzed samples in different lines (**Figure 3**). There are software tools that automate these operations to generate the data table, as well as the phase before the post-processing.

2.4.2.2. Standardization of the data of the ROIs Matrix

Of the ROI matrix integral values, the negative values are initially purged since they only contain noise (a ROI must have at least an integral value or a signal area that equals zero).

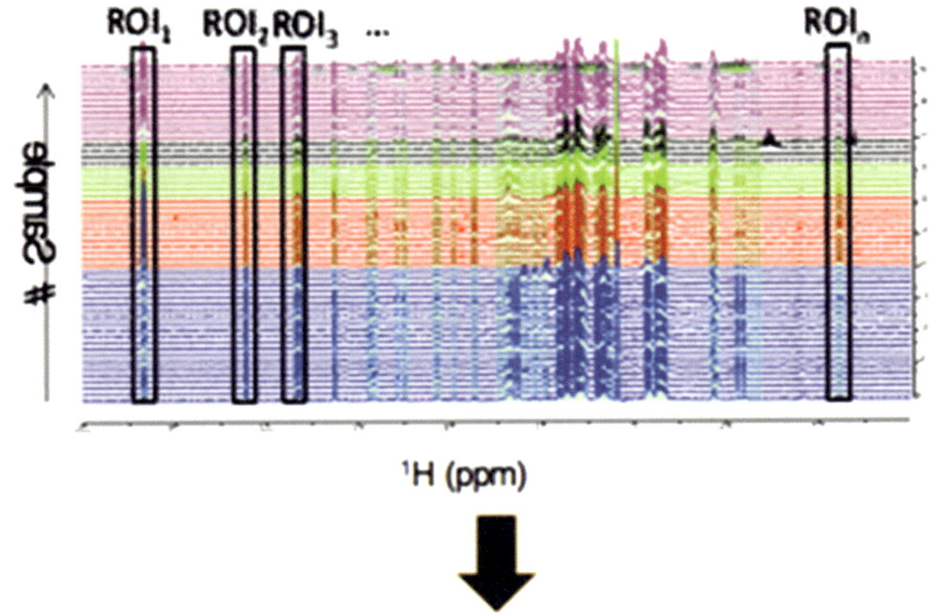

# Sample	ROI 1	ROI 2	ROI 3	...	ROI N
S1	S1_Integral1	S1_Integral2	S1_Integral3	...	S1_IntegralN
S2	S2_Integral1	S2_Integral2	S2_Integral3	...	S2_IntegralN
...	...	...	...	...	...
...	...	...	...	...	...
S53	S53_Integral1	S53_Integral2	S53_Integral3	...	S53_IntegralN

Figure 3. Scheme for the construction of a NMR ROI data matrix from 53 NMR spectra. Above: 53 ^1H spectra in which we have selected certain ROIs for the integration of the signal. The vertical piling scale identifies each of the samples (# sample). The same color has been used to identify samples that should be, a priori, of the same type. Below: NMR ROIs data matrix obtained through the integration of each of the ROIs.

The ROIs data standardization process seeks to take all the analyzed samples to a "virtual" constant that eliminates all the differences in global concentration in the ROI integral samples, which could simply respond to the urine having a higher or lower concentration of H_2O. When the dilution effect is eliminated, the differences between values of the same ROI in a pair of samples directly reflect variations in the relative concentration of the studied metabolite.

2.4.2.2.1. Standardization method of each ROI line at a standard addition

A first standardization method consists of standardizing the total addition of the ROIs. This method considers that the total addition of all the ROIs of the same spectrum has a constant value, and that this is the same for all the samples. This type of standardization by matrix lines consists of dividing each ROI value by the total addition of ROIs of its same line. As a result, the standardized ROIs of a sample add up to the unit.

2.4.2.2.2. *Probabilistic quotient standardization method*

This method consists of using the data of the ROIs of a certain sample of the study (a line of the matrix) and dividing the ROIs between those of another sample that is used as reference. This allows us to deduce the most probable multiplication factor so that the ROIs of the first sample are as close as possible to the reference sample. The most probable multiplication factor is calculated for each sample (for each line of the matrix). As a result of applying each factor on the ROIs of the relevant samples, their ROIs will be standardized as if the sample would have been prepared in the same concentration as the reference sample [115].

2.4.2.3. *Statistical analysis of the NMR ROIs Matrix*

The Matrix of standardized ROIs is analyzed by multivariate statistic methods to identify the ROIs that contain similar or different patterns of the integral in samples of the same or different group and their potential biomarkers. To do this, algorithms, such as the Principal Components Analysis (PCA), Discriminant Analysis (DA) and Orthogonal Projections to Latent Structures-Discriminant Analysis (OPLS-DA) are used. These algorithms have been implemented in several general statistical software packages, for example, R, SPSS or XLSLAT, among others.

In favorable cases, one or more ROIs with potential biomarkers related to the property under investigation are identified, for example, the effect of certain medical treatments, a type of diet, a disease, etc. Additional objectives can then be included in the study, such as the identification of what specific biomarkers (metabolites) were altered compared to the control group, to try to discover through which metabolic pathway they underwent this change. Some of the biomarkers that are identified as different from the control group may not correspond to any of those that are typically found in the relevant type of biofluid, but they may proceed from the metabolism of a drug or a special diet that has been prescribed. In this case, once its NMR signal has been identified, we could consider performing a longitudinal follow-up on its appearance in the biofluid since its administration.

2.5. Medication-related osteonecrosis of the jaw (MRONJ)

Currently, two types of drugs, aside from bisphosphonates, have been proven to cause necrosis of the jaws.

2.5.1. *Antireabsorptives: denosumab*

It is a RANKL monoclonal antibody that is currently still undergoing clinical trials for the treatment of osteoporosis, primary and metastatic bone cancer, giant cell tumor and rheumatoid arthritis [116, 117]. RANKL is necessary for the activation and function of mature osteoclasts [118, 119], which together with osteoprotegerin (OPG), maintains the balance of bone resorption in a healthy state. When an imbalance occurs in the RANKL/OPG ratio, resorption is favored in bone diseases [120, 121].

Denosumab has a high specificity due to human IgG2 that binds specifically to human RAN, and not other members of the TNF superfamily [116, 122, 123]. In clinical trials, this drug causes rapid and prolonged decreases in bone exchange markers without any change in bone formation, which gives it antireabsorptives characteristics [124]. It has also shown better clinical results compared to bisphosphonates in the treatment of osteoporosis and cancer with a higher increase in bone density and suppression of bone remodeling markers, with a proven efficacy even in patients who had been previously resistant to bisphosphonates [117, 125, 126].

These drugs also produce osteonecrosis of the jaws with a prevalence of 0.7–19% [127, 128], which is very similar to the osteonecrosis from bisphosphonate treatments [117]. Since the first case of maxillary osteonecrosis due to this drug published in 2010 [129], several studies have been published but only one of them describes histopathologic characteristics [130]. The fragments of necrotic bone showed empty osteocytic lacuna and absence of osteocytes, osteoblasts and osteoclasts. The authors suggest that these characteristics are very similar to bisphosphonate-related osteonecrosis [131]

2.5.2. Antiangiogenics

These drugs hinder the development of new blood vessels and block the cascade of angiogenesis [132].

Bevacizumab: Monoclonal antibodies that stop the growth factor.

Suntinib and Sorafenib: Tyrosine kinase inhibitors.

3. Results of our experience

3.1. Regarding the risk factors

All the patients of this study visited the Master of Oral Medicine, Surgery and Implantology of the Faculty of Dentistry of the University of Santiago de Compostela. The patients were derived from the Unit of Oncology of the Complejo Hospitalario Universitario de Santiago de Compostela (CHUS) for a dental examination prior to treatment with intravenous bisphosphonates. The study was approved by the Clinical Research Ethics Committee of Galicia, in addition to the gaining informed consent from the patients.

Patients treated with zoledronic acid for a period of 7 years (2006–2013) and patients with a history of treatment of head and neck radiotherapy were excluded.

Local risk factors: Only those patients who underwent exodontics during bisphosphonate treatment had a statistically significant risk ($P > 0.001$), as well as a direct relationship according to the periodontal status of the patient, since no patient with periodontal health developed MRONJ ($P = 0.001$). As previously described in the literature, research showed that the mandible is more affected than the upper maxilla and is also statistically significant ($P < 0.001$)

Systemic risk factors: There were no significant differences in terms of gender ($P = 0.063$). Age did not show significant differences but there were more cases of osteonecrosis in elderly patients, probably because these patients are more compromised at the systemic level; in fact,

86.6% of them were polymedicated. The type of cancer, arterial hypertension and treatment with chemotherapy or corticosteroids did not show statistically significant differences, although the literature describes them as obvious risk factors. We could only conclude that patients without diabetes did not develop MRONJ (P = 0.048). In our study we did not factor in their race, since 100% of the patients were Caucasian and from a specific population. As described by Wessel et al. [29] in their study, 100% of our patients had bone metastases, which justified the use of intravenous bisphosphonates and, therefore, also implied an increased risk of complications.

Drug-related factors: Regarding potency, all patients were treated with the same bisphosphonate (zoledronic acid, 4 mg). The cumulative dose showed that patients with more than three years of treatment had a higher risk of developing MRONJ, which was statistically significant (P < 0.001) (**Table 5**).

3.2. Bacterial role in osteonecrosis of the jaws

We selected 28 patients (16 men and 12 women) with a mean age of 71.96 years, all of whom were treated in the Oncology Department of the Complejo Hospitalario Universitario de Santiago de Compostela (CHUS). They were referred to the Unit of Oral Surgery and Implantology of the Faculty of Medicine and Dentistry of Santiago de Compostela for a prior dental examination and for the follow-up of possible complications after treatment.

All patients treated with both oral and intravenous bisphosphonates and those undergoing head and neck radiotherapy within an 8-year period were included (2006–2014). The diagnostic criteria followed were those determined by the AAOMS [15] for patients treated with bisphosphonates, while in the case of those undergoing radiotherapy, we included those who had bone exposure for more than 8 weeks.

Samples of exudates from bone exposure were sent to the Department of Microbiology to be processed under Gram staining and seeded in liquid medium (thioglycolate broth) and in solids (agar-blood and agar-chocolate for the growth of aerobic bacteria, Sabouraud agar for yeast growth and Schaedler agar for anaerobic growth). The seeded plates were incubated for 48 h at 37°C in a CO_2 atmosphere and 72 h in anaerobic chambers. Identification of microorganisms was done using the Vitek 2 system (Bio-Merieux, Marcy l'Etoile, France) and Microscam (Siemens, Erlangen, Germany) in the case of aerobes; and API-ANA (Biomeriex) in the case of anaerobes. Antimicrobial susceptibility testing was performed by the e-test method (AB biodisk) and the Clinical Laboratory Standards Institute (CLSI) interpretation criteria were followed.

Biopsies of bone sequestration were sent to the Pathological Anatomy Service where they were fixed in 10% buffered formaldehyde and embedded in paraffin following standard processing. For evaluation, they were stained with hematoxylin/eosin, PAS and methenamine silver to visualize the colonies of Actinomyces. Their presence was evaluated semi-quantitatively and divided into scarce, moderately abundant or very abundant. In addition, the presence of acute inflammation (when polymorphonuclear neutrophil cells were observed), which was also quantified in three degrees: mild, moderate and intense, and the presence of chronic inflammation (indicated by the presence of lymphocytes and plasma cells).

Characteristics	Total patients with ONJ (%)	Total patients without ONJ (%)	P
Gender			0.063
Men	14 (7.2)	125 (64.4)	
Women	11 (5.7)	44 (22.7)	
Systemic Risk Factor			0.214
Cancer	12 (6.2)	95 (49)	
Prostate	9 (4.6)	34 (17.5)	
Breast	4 (2)	11 (5.7)	
Myeloma	0 (0)	18 (9.3)	
Lung	0 (0)	2 (1)	
Bladder	0 (0)	5 (2.6)	
Colon	0 (0)	3 (1.5)	
Kidney	18 (9.3)	176 (90.7)	
Diabetes	168 (86.6)	26 (13.4)	0.048
Polymedicated.	94 (48.5)	100 (51.5)	0.139
HTA	42 (21.6)	152 (78.4)	0.704
Cortisone	65 (33.5)	129 (66.5)	0.234
QTP	11 (5.7)	54 (27.8)	0.462
Local Risk Factor			
Extraction Before	8 (4.1)	86 (44.3)	0.078
Extraction during	5 (2.6)	1 (0.5)	<0.001
Extraction after	4 (2)	7 (3.6)	0.017
Prosthesis	5 (2.6)	33 (17)	0.936
periodontal state	19 (9.8)	70 (36)	0.001
Toxic factors			0.998
Tobacco	2 (1)	13 (6.7)	
Alcohol	3 (1.5)	19 (9.8)	
Location			
Unifocal mandible	13 (6.7)	–	<0.001
Unifocal maxilla	5 (2.6)	–	
Multifocal mandible	3 (1.5)	–	
Maxilla and mandible	4 (2)	–	

Table 5. Risk factors in the occurrence of ONJ.

The collected data were analyzed with the SPSS statistical system, version 20.0 for Windows. The discontinuous quantitative or discreet variables were analyzed through descriptive statistics, expressing the results in mean, deviation and standard. The frequency tables and percentages were used for qualitative variables. For the study of the association of variables we employed the chi-squared test, the T-Student test or the ANOVA factor test, depending on the application conditions. Values in which $P \leq 0.05$ were considered statistically significant.

3.2.1. *Clinical results*

Of the 28 patients, 16 were men (57.1%) and 12 women (48.8%) with a mean age of 71.96 years (SD 8.94). According to the risk factors analyzed, 8 patients (28.5%) were diabetic, 15 (53.6%) were undergoing chemotherapy, 4 were smokers (14.3%), 14 was hypertensive (50%) and 9 (32.1%) were taking corticosteroids. The reason for treatment with bisphosphonates was oral cancer (14.3%), breast cancer (25%), prostate cancer (39.2%), multiple myeloma (10.7%) and osteoporosis (10.7%).

The most affected region of the mouth was the mandible (67.8%) followed by the upper jaw (21.4%) or both (10.7%).

The degree of affectation was variable depending on the type of treatment. Patients on intravenous bisphosphonates had all stages of ONJ, whereas patients undergoing the oral treatment had only stage II ONJ and patients treated with radiotherapy showed both stage II (5%) and stage III (75%).

3.2.2. *Histological results*

A total of 24 of 28 patients underwent a histological study with a biopsy of a bone sequestration lesion. Of these, in 21 patients (87.5%) we proved the presence of Actinomyces within the 3 degrees of osteonecrosis of the jaws. The amount of Actinomyces present was quantified semi-quantitatively by the pathologist. The pathogen count was very abundant in degrees I and II, while in degree III the patients had lower amounts of Actinomyces (**Figure 4**).

The degree of acute and/or chronic inflammation was also evaluated. In 54.2% of the patients, the presence of Actinomyces was not accompanied by any sign of inflammation; while in the rest of the patients, it was observed that as age increased, the intensity of the inflammation also increased; therefore a lower mean age accounted for the absence of inflammation (65.31; SD: 7.91) contrasting with abundant inflammation (81.00; SD: 2.83). Such differences were statistically significant ($F = 5.270$, $P = 0.005$). There was acute inflammation in 37.5% of the patients being quantified as mild inflammation (two patients), moderate (five patients) and severe (two patients); the latter two were present in patients with grade II osteonecrosis, exclusively. There were only two chronic inflammation cases, one patient with grade II and another with grade III ONJ.

The relationship between the amount of Actinomyces present in the histological sections and the degree of inflammation observed in bone sequestration was evaluated. Despite not having statistically significant data, it was observed that the high amount of Actinomyces could trigger either null or an abundant inflammatory response (**Table 6**).

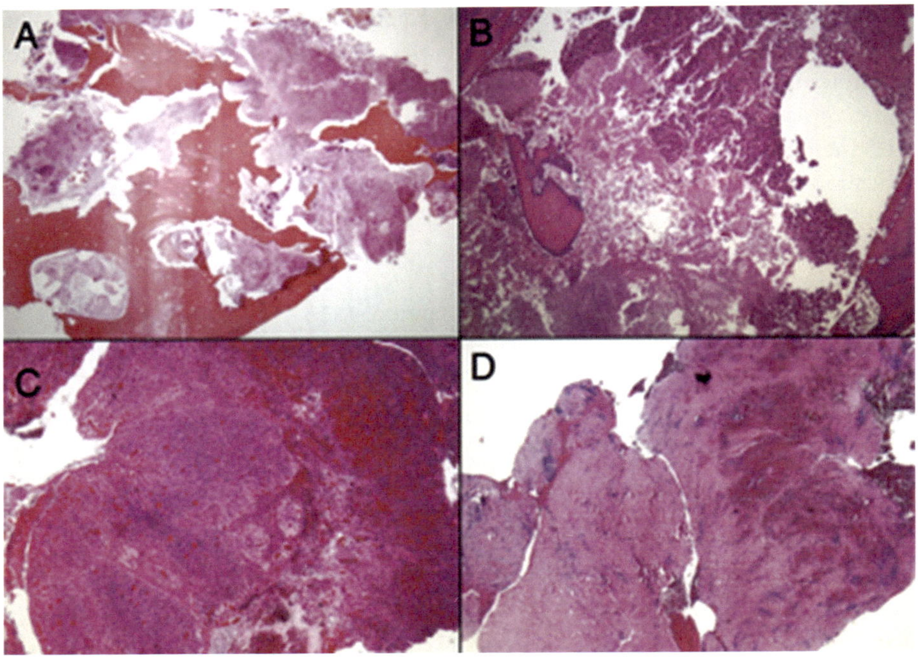

Figure 4. Histological image of bone sequestration. Histopathologic examination revealed different combinations of Actinomyces and the inflammatory response. Some cases showed abundant colonies of Actinomyces, but lacked any inflammatory infiltration (A); while in other examples this microorganism was identified along with a dense PMN infiltrate (B). PMNs were also seen in some cases, in the absence of Actinomyces (C). Last of all, in some patients, the only change consisted of fibrosis and the scarce inflammatory response was composed mainly of lymphocytes (D).

3.2.3. Microbiological results

Regarding the isolation of bacteria obtained through suppuration of the necrosed area, all the bacteria described by the microbiologist were recorded, which were later classified according to their aerobic or anaerobic metabolism. Aerobic bacteria were mostly found (85%) in patients with grade I and II of ONJ, being statistically significant (P = 0.002). However, anaerobic bacteria were present in 56% of the patients in the three stages of ONJ. Although all the cases of grade III presented anaerobic bacteria, this data were not statistically significant.

	Inflammation				
Actinomyces	**Null**	**Mild**	**Moderate**	**Abundant**	**Chronic**
Null	0	0	1	0	0
Scarce	1	0	1	0	1
Moderate	8	1	1	0	1
Abundant	4	1	2	2	0

Table 6. Relationship of the amount of Actinomyces and the inflammatory response.

There was practically no significance in the families of bacterial species specific to the different degrees of osteonecrosis, except *Streptococcus* sp. which was very abundant in grade II of ONJ. Only three bacteria showed statistically significant differences in relation to the ONJ stages (**Table 7**, **Figure 5**).

Antibiograms were also performed for each of the species found, in order to guide the antibiotic pattern of these patients. We studied the six most common antibiotics, as well as the specific ones for the pathology described in the literature, we observed a variable bacterial behavior among the patients with osteonecrosis of the jaws.

Penicillin G did not show complete sensitivity in any patient against all the bacteria isolated in the cultures, in addition, there was much variability among patients regarding the response to this antibiotic (**Figure 6**).

The combination of amoxicillin and clavulanic acid showed good sensitivity in most patients (82.6%) although this was not statistically significant (**Figure 7**).

Clindamycin was effective in 40% of patients and resistant in 14.5%, while 28% of the patients showed variability in the response to this antibiotic. Azithromycin was effective in a few patients (38%) and the response was highly variable, without showing complete sensitivity to isolated bacteria (**Figure 8**).

Levofloxacin was effective in 42.8% of the patients, which showed good sensitivity in most cases (88.8%). Last of all, gentamicin, another antibiotic which is less frequent in our daily practice, showed good sensitivity although it was effective in few patients (38%).

	Grade I	Grade II	Grade III	P value
Staphylococcus sp.	0	1	1	0.372
Capnocytophaga sp.	2	1	0	0.008
Morganella morganii	0	1	0	0.817
Enterobacter cloacae	0	1	2	0.037
Streptococcus sp.	3	12	1	0.112
Eikenella corrodens	0	3	1	0.664
Neisseria sp.	3	3	0	0.004
Proteus sp.	0	1	0	0.074
Actinomyces sp.	2	3	0	0.003
Veionella parvula	0	0	2	0.817
Peptostreptococcus sp.	0	3	0	0.515
Fusobacterium sp.	0	1	1	0.372
Prevotella sp.	0	4	1	0.648
Bacteroides sp.	0	2	0	0.655

Table 7. Relationship between the isolated type of bacteria and the degree of ONJ.

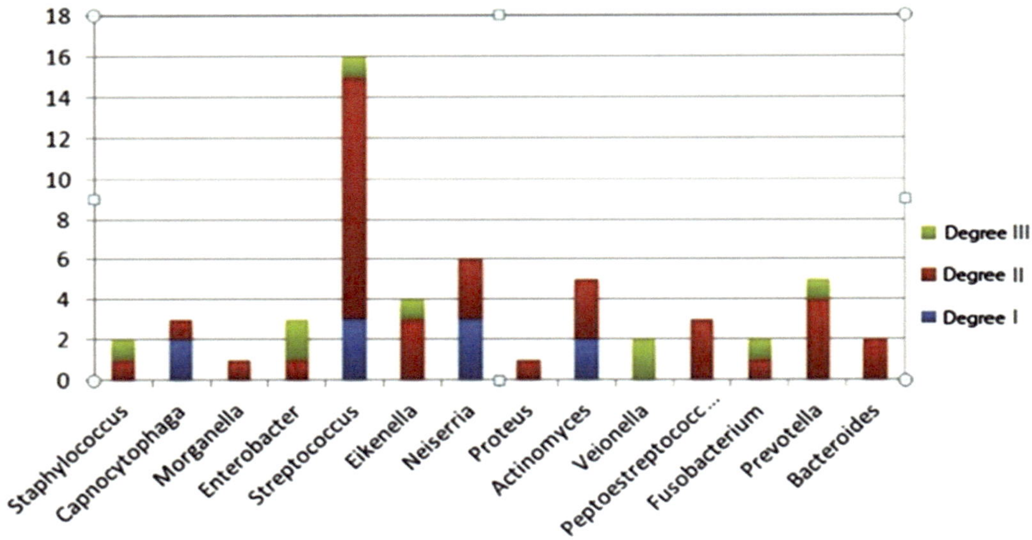

Figure 5. Relationship between the isolated type of bacteria and the degree of ONJ.

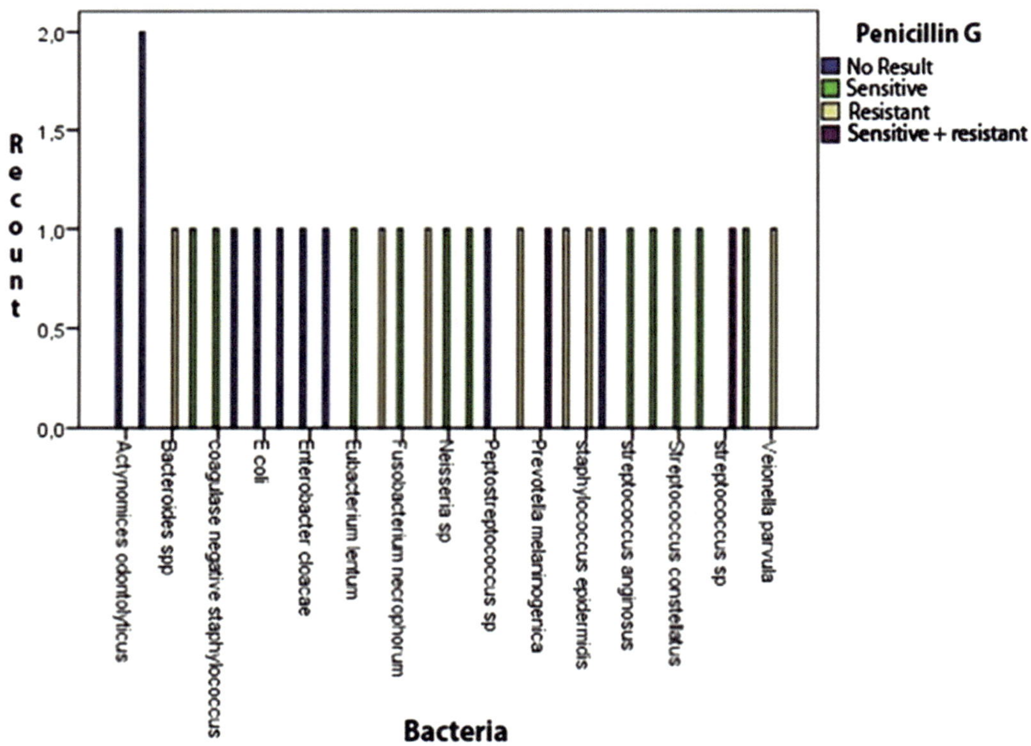

Figure 6. Antibiogram of Penicillin G.

http://dx.doi.org/10.5772/intechopen.69315

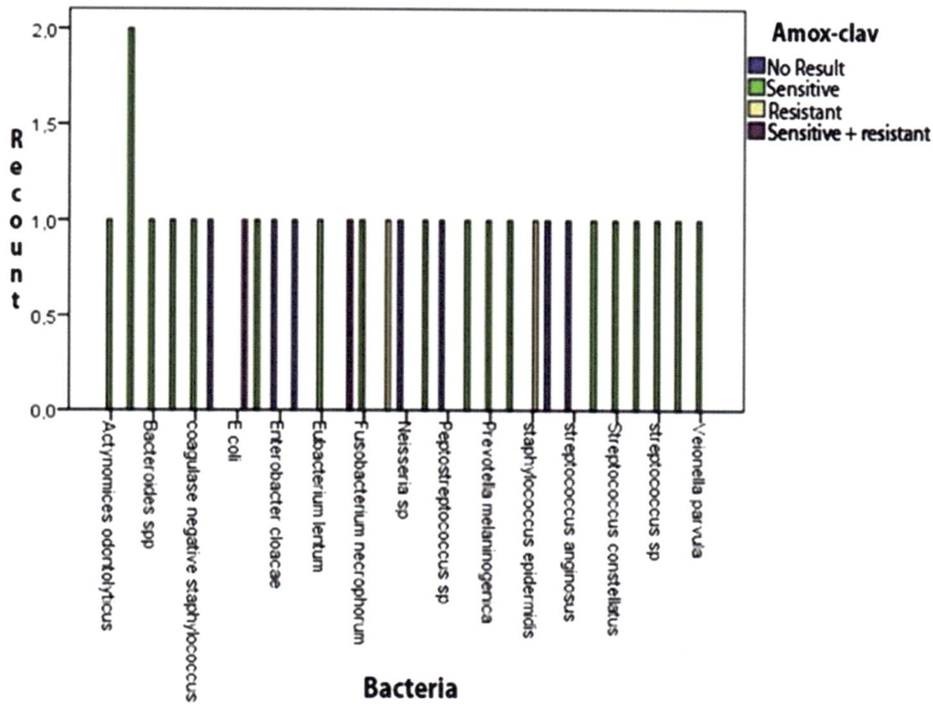

Figure 7. Antibiogram of the association of amoxicillin with clavulanic acid.

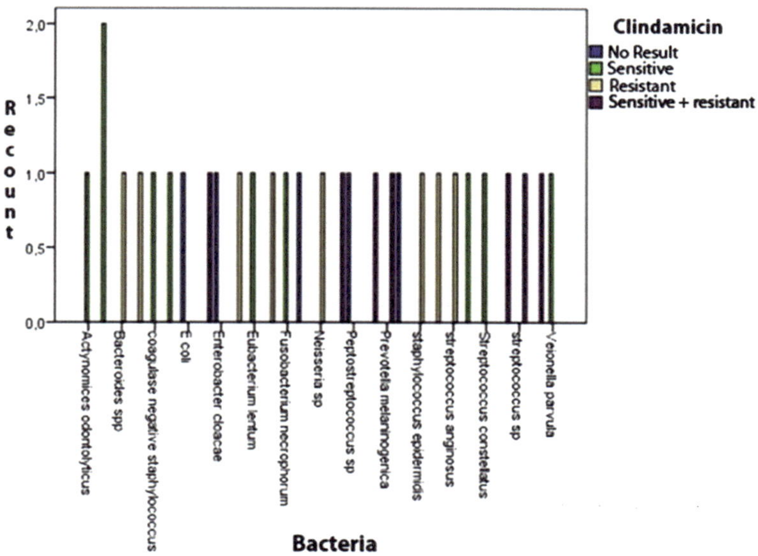

Figure 8. Clindamycin antibiogram.

Acknowledgement

I would like to thank to Aram Ríos for his invaluable cooperation in graphic design of the book chapter.

Author details

Mario Pérez-Sayáns[1]*, Carmen Vidal-Real[1], José M. Suárez-Peñaranda[2] and Abel García-García[1]

*Address all correspondence to: perezsayans@gmail.com

1 Oral Medicine, Oral Surgery and Implantology Unit, Faculty of Medicine and Dentistry, Instituto de Investigación Sanitaria de Santiago (IDIS), Santiago de Compostela, Spain

2 Servicio de Anatomía Patológica, Hospital Clínica Universitario de Santiago, Spain

References

[1] Lapidus FI. Cancer and osteonecrosis of the lower jaw following irradiation. Stomatologiia (Mosk). 1950;**2**:34-36

[2] Gowgiel JM. Experimental radio-osteonecrosis of the jaws. Journal of Dental Research. 1960 Jan-Feb;**39**:176-197

[3] Lawrence EA. Osteoradionecrosis of the mandible. The American Journal of Roentgenology and Radium Therapy. 1946 Jun;**55**:733-742

[4] Gallagher RE. Arsenic—new life for an old potion. New England Journal of Medicine. 1998;**339**(19):1389-1391

[5] Cruse WP, Bellizzi R. A historic review of endodontics, 1689-1963, part 1. Journal of Endodontics. 1980;**6**(3):495-499

[6] Dumlu A, Yalcinkaya S, Olgac V, Güvercin M. Osteomyelitis due to arsenic trioxide use for tooth devitalization. International Endodontic Journal. 2007;**40**(4):317-322

[7] Tal M, Kaufman A, Buchner A. Bone necrosis and dentine resorption caused by Toxavit: A case report. International Endodontic Journal. 1978;**11**(2):77-79

[8] Bataineh A, Al-Omari M, Owais A. Arsenical necrosis of the jaws. International Endodontic Journal. 1997;**30**(4):283-287

[9] Sanders B, McKelvy B, Adams D. Aseptic osteomyelitis and necrosis of the mandibular condylar head after intracapsular fracture. Oral Surgery, Oral Medicine, and Oral Pathology. 1977;**43**(5):665-670

[10] Lanigan DT, West RA. Aseptic necrosis of the mandible: Report of two cases. Journal of Oral and Maxillofacial Surgery. 1990;**48**(3):296-300

[11] Sung EC, Chan SM, Sakurai K, Chung E. Osteonecrosis of the maxilla as a complication to chemotherapy: A case report. Special Care in Dentistry. 2002;**22**(4):142-146

[12] Marx RE. Pamidronate (Aredia) and zoledronate (Zometa) induced avascular necrosis of the jaws: A growing epidemic. Journal of Oral and Maxillofacial Surgery. 2003 Sep;**61**(9):1115-1117

[13] Gupta S, Jain P, Kumar P, Parikh PM. Zoledronic acid induced osteonecrosis of tibia and femur. Indian Journal of Cancer. 2009 Jul-Sep;**46**(3):249-250

[14] Polizzotto MN, Cousins V, Schwarer AP. Bisphosphonate-associated osteonecrosis of the auditory canal. British Journal of Haematology. 2006;**132**(1):114-114

[15] Advisory Task Force on Bisphosphonate-Related Ostenonecrosis of the Jaws, American Association of Oral and Maxillofacial Surgeons. American Association of Oral and Maxillofacial Surgeons position paper on bisphosphonate-related osteonecrosis of the jaws. Journal of Oral and Maxillofacial Surgery. 2007 Mar;**65**(3):369-376

[16] Ruggiero SL, Dodson TB, Assael LA, Landesberg R, Marx RE, Mehrotra B, et al. American Association of Oral and Maxillofacial Surgeons position paper on bisphosphonate-related osteonecrosis of the jaw - 2009 update. Australian Endodontic Journal. 2009 Dec;**35**(3):119-130

[17] Ruggiero SL, Dodson TB, Fantasia J, Goodday R, Aghaloo T, Mehrotra B, et al. American Association of Oral and Maxillofacial Surgeons position paper on medication-related osteonecrosis of the jaw—2014 update. Journal of Oral and Maxillofacial Surgery. 2014;**72**(10):1938-1956

[18] Khan A, Morrison A, Cheung A, Hashem W, Compston J. Osteonecrosis of the jaw (ONJ): Diagnosis and management in 2015. Osteoporosis International. 2016;**27**(3):853-859

[19] Ruggiero SL, Dodson TB, Assael LA, Landesberg R, Marx RE, Mehrotra B. American Association of Oral and Maxillofacial Surgeons position paper on bisphosphonate-related osteonecrosis of the jaws—2009 update. Journal of Oral and Maxillofacial Surgery. 2009;**67**(5):2-12

[20] IMS HEALTH. NPA Plus™; May 2006

[21] American Dental Association. Report of the Council of Scientific Affairs. Expert Panel Recommendations: Dental Management of Patients on Oral Bisphosphonate Therapy. June 2006. [Cited 29 Jun 2006.] Available from URL: http://www.ada.org/prof/resources/topics/osteonecrosis.asp

[22] Mavrokokki T, Cheng A, Stein B, Goss A. Nature and frequency of bisphosphonate-associated osteonecrosis of the jaws in Australia. Journal of Oral and Maxillofacial Surgery. 2007;**65**(3):415-423

[23] Ault A. Jaw necrosis affects 1 in 1,700 on oral bisphosphonates. Internal Medicine News. 2008;**41**(15):23-23

[24] Ruggiero SL, Fantasia J, Carlson E. Bisphosphonate-related osteonecrosis of the jaw: Background and guidelines for diagnosis, staging and management. Oral Surgery, Oral Medicine, Oral Pathology, Oral Radiology, and Endodontics. 2006;**102**(4):433-441

[25] Ruggiero SL, Mehrotra B, Rosenberg TJ, Engroff SL. Osteonecrosis of the jaws associated with the use of bisphosphonates: A review of 63 cases. Journal of Oral and Maxillofacial Surgery. 2004 May;**62**(5):527-534

[26] Marx RE, Sawatari Y, Fortin M, Broumand V. Bisphosphonate-induced exposed bone (osteonecrosis/osteopetrosis) of the jaws: Risk factors, recognition, prevention, and treatment. Journal of Oral and Maxillofacial Surgery. 2005 Nov;**63**(11):1567-1575

[27] Hoff, AO, Toth, BB, Altundag, K, Guarneri, V, Adamus, A, Nooka, AK, Sayegh GG, Johnson MM, Gagel RF & Hortobagyi GN. Osteonecrosis of the jaw in patients receiving intravenous bisphosphonate therapy. Journal of Clinical Oncology. 2006;**24**(90180):8528-8528

[28] Badros A, Weikel D, Salama A, Goloubeva O, Schneider A, Rapoport A, et al. Osteonecrosis of the jaw in multiple myeloma patients: Clinical features and risk factors. Journal of Clinical Oncology. 2006 Feb 20;**24**(6):945-952

[29] Wessel JH, Dodson TB, Zavras AI. Zoledronate, smoking, and obesity are strong risk factors for osteonecrosis of the jaw: A case-control study. Journal of Oral and Maxillofacial Surgery. 2008;**66**(4):625-631

[30] Zervas K, Verrou E, Teleioudis Z, Vahtsevanos K, Banti A, Mihou D, et al. Incidence, risk factors and management of osteonecrosis of the jaw in patients with multiple myeloma: A single-centre experience in 303 patients. British Journal of Haematology. 2006;**134**(6):620-623

[31] Jadu F, Lee L, Pharoah M, Reece D, Wang L. A retrospective study assessing the incidence, risk factors and comorbidities of pamidronate-related necrosis of the jaws in multiple myeloma patients. Annals of Oncology. 2007 Dec;**18**(12):2015-2019

[32] Hoefert S, Schmitz I, Tannapfel A, Eufinger H. Importance of microcracks in etiology of bisphosphonate-related osteonecrosis of the jaw: A possible pathogenetic model of symptomatic and non-symptomatic osteonecrosis of the jaw based on scanning electron microscopy findings. Clinical Oral Investigations. 2010;**14**(3):271-284

[33] English BC, Baum CE, Adelberg DE, Sissung TM, Kluetz PG, Dahut WL, et al. A SNP in CYP2C8 is not associated with the development of bisphosphonate-related osteonecrosis of the jaw in men with castrate-resistant prostate cancer. Therapeutics and Clinical Risk Management. 2010 Nov 19;**6**:579-583

[34] Sarasquete ME, Garcia-Sanz R, Marin L, Alcoceba M, Chillon MC, Balanzategui A, et al. Bisphosphonate-related osteonecrosis of the jaw is associated with polymorphisms of the cytochrome P450 CYP2C8 in multiple myeloma: A genome-wide single nucleotide polymorphism analysis. Blood. 2008 Oct 1;**112**(7):2709-2712.

[35] Khamaisi M, Regev E, Yarom N, Avni B, Leitersdorf E, Raz I, et al. Possible association between diabetes and bisphosphonate-related jaw osteonecrosis. The Journal of Clinical Endocrinology & Metabolism. 2007;**92**(3):1172-1175

[36] Bedogni A, Fusco V, Agrillo A, Campisi G. Learning from experience. Proposal of a refined definition and staging system for bisphosphonate-related osteonecrosis of the jaw (BRONJ). Oral Diseases. 2012;**18**(6):621-623

[37] Fedele S, Porter SR, D'Aiuto F, Aljohani S, Vescovi P, Manfredi M, et al. Nonexposed variant of bisphosphonate-associated osteonecrosis of the jaw: A case series. American Journal of Medicine. 2010;**123**(11):1060-1064

[38] Arce K, Assael LA, Weissman JL, Markiewicz MR. Imaging findings in bisphosphonate-related osteonecrosis of jaws. Journal of Oral and Maxillofacial Surgery. 2009;**67**(5):75-84

[39] Ruggiero SL. Guidelines for the diagnosis of bisphosphonate-related osteonecrosis of the jaw (BRONJ). Clinical Cases in Mineral and Bone Metabolism. 2007;**4**(1):37

[40] Mawardi H, Giro G, Kajiya M, Ohta K, Almazrooa S, Alshwaimi E, et al. A role of oral bacteria in bisphosphonate-induced osteonecrosis of the jaw. Journal of Dental Research. 2011 Nov;**90**(11):1339-1345

[41] Katsarelis H, Shah NP, Dhariwal DK, Pazianas M. Infection and medication-related osteonecrosis of the jaw. Journal of Dental Research. 2015 Apr;**94**(4):534-539

[42] Wimalawansa SJ. Insight into bisphosphonate-associated osteomyelitis of the jaw: Pathophysiology, mechanisms and clinical management. Expert Opinion on Drug Safety. 2008;**7**(4):491-512

[43] Allen MR, Burr DB. The pathogenesis of bisphosphonate-related osteonecrosis of the jaw: So many hypotheses, so few data. Journal of Oral and Maxillofacial Surgery. 2009 May;**67**(5 Suppl):61-70

[44] Lee CY, Pien FD, Suzuki JB. Identification and treatment of bisphosphonate-associated actinomycotic osteonecrosis of the jaws. Implant Dentistry. 2011 Oct;**20**(5):331-336

[45] Schipmann S, Metzler P, Rossle M, Zemann W, von Jackowski J, Obwegeser JA, et al. Osteopathology associated with bone resorption inhibitors - which role does Actinomyces play? A presentation of 51 cases with systematic review of the literature. Journal of Oral Pathology and Medicine. 2013 Sep;**42**(8):587-593

[46] De Ceulaer J, Tacconelli E, Vandecasteele S. Actinomyces osteomyelitis in bisphosphonate-related osteonecrosis of the jaw (BRONJ): The missing link?. European Journal of Clinical Microbiology & Infectious Diseases. 2014;**33**(11):1873-1880

[47] Moghimi M, Salentijn E, Debets Ossenkop Y, Karagozoglu KH, & Forouzanfar T. Treatment of cervicofacial actinomycosis: A report of 19 cases and review of literature. Medicina Oral, Patología Oral y Cirugía Bucal. 2013 Jul 1;**18**(4):e627–e632

[48] Steininger C, Willinger B. Resistance patterns in clinical isolates of pathogenic Actinomyces species. Journal of Antimicrobial Chemotherapy. 2016 Feb;**71**(2):422-427

[49] Bocci V. Ozone as Janus: This controversial gas can be either toxic or medically useful. Mediators of Inflammation. 2004 Feb;**13**(1):3-11

[50] Ripamonti CI, Cislaghi E, Mariani L, Maniezzo M. Efficacy and safety of medical ozone (O3) delivered in oil suspension applications for the treatment of osteonecrosis of the jaw in patients with bone metastases treated with bisphosphonates: Preliminary results of a phase I–II study. Oral Oncology. 2011;**47**(3):185-190

[51] Vescovi P, Manfredi M, Merigo E, Meleti M, Fornaini C, Rocca J, et al. Surgical approach with Er: YAG laser on osteonecrosis of the jaws (ONJ) in patients under bisphosphonate therapy (BPT). Lasers in Medical Science. 2010;**25**(1):101-113

[52] Vescovi P, Merigo E, Meleti M, Manfredi M, Fornaini C, Nammour S, et al. Conservative surgical management of stage I bisphosphonate-related osteonecrosis of the jaw. International Journal of Dentistry. 2014;**2014**:107690

[53] Freiberger JJ, Padilla-Burgos R, McGraw T, Suliman HB, Kraft KH, Stolp BW, et al. What is the role of hyperbaric oxygen in the management of bisphosphonate-related osteonecrosis of the jaw: A randomized controlled trial of hyperbaric oxygen as an adjunct to surgery and antibiotics. Journal of Oral and Maxillofacial Surgery. 2012;**70**(7):1573-1583

[54] Atalay B, Yalcin S, Emes Y, Aktas I, Aybar B, Issever H, et al. Bisphosphonate-related osteonecrosis: Laser-assisted surgical treatment or conventional surgery?. Lasers in Medical Science. 2011;**26**(6):815-823

[55] Rodriguez-Lozano, FJ, & Oñate-Sánchez, RE. Treatment of osteonecrosis of the jaw related to bisphosphonates and other antiresorptive agents. Medicina Oral, Patología Oral y Cirugía Bucal. 2016;**21**(5):e595

[56] Bedogni A, Saia G, Bettini G, Tronchet A, Totola A, Bedogni G, et al. Long-term outcomes of surgical resection of the jaws in cancer patients with bisphosphonate-related osteonecrosis. Oral Oncology. 2011;**47**(5):420-424

[57] Schubert M, Klatte I, Linek W, Müller B, Döring K, Eckelt U, et al. The Saxon Bisphosphonate Register–Therapy and prevention of bisphosphonate-related osteonecrosis of the jaws. Oral Oncology. 2012;**48**(4):349-354

[58] Cella L, Oppici A, Arbasi M, Moretto M, Piepoli M, Vallisa D, et al. Autologous bone marrow stem cell intralesional transplantation repairing bisphosphonate related osteonecrosis of the jaw. Head & Face Medicine. 2011;**7**(1):1

[59] Gonzalvez-Garcia M, Rodriguez-Lozano FJ, Villanueva V, Segarra-Fenoll D, Rodriguez-Gonzalez MA, Onate-Sanchez R, et al. Cell therapy in bisphosphonate-related osteonecrosis of the jaw. The Journal of Craniofacial Surgery. 2013 May;**24**(3):e226–e228

[60] Curi MM, Cossolin GSI, Koga DH, Zardetto C, Christianini S, Feher O, et al. Bisphosphonate-related osteonecrosis of the jaws–an initial case series report of treatment combining partial bone resection and autologous platelet-rich plasma. Journal of Oral and Maxillofacial Surgery. 2011;**69**(9):2465-2472

[61] Cheung A, Seeman E. Teriparatide therapy for alendronate-associated osteonecrosis of the jaw. New England Journal of Medicine. 2010;**363**(25):2473-2474

[62] Kim J, Kim S, Kim M. Leucocyte-rich and platelet-rich fibrin for the treatment of bisphosphonate-related osteonecrosis of the jaw: A prospective feasibility study. British Journal of Oral and Maxillofacial Surgery. 2014;**52**(9):854-859

[63] Dimopoulos MA, Kastritis E, Bamia C, Melakopoulos I, Gika D, Roussou M, et al. Reduction of osteonecrosis of the jaw (ONJ) after implementation of preventive measures in patients with multiple myeloma treated with zoledronic acid. Annals of Oncology. 2009 Jan;**20**(1):117-120

[64] Mehrotra, B., Fantasia, J, & Ruggiero, SL. Outcomes of bisphosphonate-related osteonecrosis of the jaw—Importance of staging and management guidelines: A large single institutional update. Journal of Clinical Oncology. 2008;**26**(90150):20526-20526

[65] Corso A, Varettoni M, Zappasodi P, Klersy C, Mangiacavalli S, Pica G, et al. A different schedule of zoledronic acid can reduce the risk of the osteonecrosis of the jaw in patients with multiple myeloma. Leukemia. 2007;**21**(7):1545-1548

[66] Rosen H, Moses A, Garber J, Iloputaife I, Ross D, Lee S, et al. Serum CTX: A new marker of bone resorption that shows treatment effect more often than other markers because of low coefficient of variability and large changes with bisphosphonate therapy. Calcified Tissue International. 2000;**66**(2):100-103

[67] Carlson ER, Basile JD. The role of surgical resection in the management of bisphosphonate-related osteonecrosis of the jaws. Journal of Oral and Maxillofacial Surgery. 2009;**67**(5):85-95

[68] Marx RE, Cillo Jr JE, Ulloa JJ. Oral bisphosphonate-induced osteonecrosis: Risk factors, prediction of risk using serum CTX testing, prevention, and treatment. Journal of Oral and Maxillofacial Surgery. 2007;**65**(12):2397-2410

[69] Migliorati CA, Siegel MA, Elting LS. Bisphosphonate-associated osteonecrosis: A long-term complication of bisphosphonate treatment. The Lancet Oncology. 2006;**7**(6): 508-514

[70] American Association of Endodontists Position Statement. Endodontic Implications of Bisphosphonate-Associated Osteonecrosis of the Jaws. [Cited 14 Aug 2006.] RL: http://www.aae.org/dentalpro/guidelines.htm

[71] Enciso R, Keaton J, Saleh N, Ahmadieh A, Clark GT, & Sedghizadeh PP Assessing the utility of serum C-telopeptide cross-link of type 1 collagen as a predictor of bisphosphonate-related osteonecrosis of the jaw: A systematic review and meta-analysis. The Journal of the American Dental Association. 2016;**147**(7):551-560

[72] Borromeo G, Tsao C, Darby I, Ebeling P. A review of the clinical implications of bisphosphonates in dentistry. Australian Dental Journal. 2011;**56**(1):2-9

[73] Rodan GA, Fleisch HA. Bisphosphonates: Mechanisms of action. Journal of Clinical Investigation. 1996 Jun 15;**97**(12):2692-2696

[74] Wood J, Bonjean K, Ruetz S, Bellahcene A, Devy L, Foidart JM, et al. Novel antiangiogenic effects of the bisphosphonate compound zoledronic acid. Journal of Pharmacology and Experimental Therapeutics. 2002 Sep;**302**(3):1055-1061

[75] Santini D, Vincenzi B, Avvisati G, Dicuonzo G, Battistoni F, Gavasci M, et al. Pamidronate induces modifications of circulating angiogenetic factors in cancer patients. Clinical Cancer Research. 2002 May;**8**(5):1080-1084

[76] Kapitola J, Zak J, Lacinova Z, Justova V. Effect of growth hormone and pamidronate on bone blood flow, bone mineral and IGF-I levels in the rat. Physiological Research. 2000;**49**:S101–S106

[77] Kapitola J, Zak J. Effect of pamidronate on bone blood flow in oophorectomized rats. Physiological Research. 1998;**47**:237-240

[78] Fournier P, Boissier S, Filleur S, Guglielmi J, Cabon F, Colombel M, et al. Bisphosphonates inhibit angiogenesis in vitro and testosterone-stimulated vascular regrowth in the ventral prostate in castrated rats. Cancer Research. 2002 Nov 15;**62**(22):6538-6544

[79] Corso A, Ferretti E, Lunghi M, Zappasodi P, Mangiacavalli S, De Amici M, et al. Zoledronic acid down-regulates adhesion molecules of bone marrow stromal cells in multiple myeloma. Cancer. 2005;**104**(1):118-125

[80] Berenson JR, Hillner BE, Kyle RA, Anderson K, Lipton A, Yee GC, et al. American Society of Clinical Oncology clinical practice guidelines: The role of bisphosphonates in multiple myeloma. Journal of Clinical Oncology. 2002 Sep 1;**20**(17):3719-3736

[81] Physicians' Desk Reference. 57th ed. Montvale, NJ: Medical Economics; 2003

[82] Hohnecker JA. Novartis 'Dear Doctor' Precautions Added to Label of Aredia and Zometa. Novartis Pharmaceuticals Corporation East Hanover USA. September 24, 2004.

[83] Almojaly, S. The Effect of the Bisphosphonate, Alendronate, on Primary Human Alveolar Bone Cells. State University of New York at Buffalo, ProQuest Dissertations Publishing; Paris, France. 2008. 1453398

[84] http://www.fda.gov/ohms/dockets/ac/05/briefing/2005-4095b1.htm

[85] Green JR, Müller K, Jaeggi KA. Preclinical pharmacology of CGP 42′ 446, a new, potent, heterocyclic bisphosphonate compound. Journal of Bone and Mineral Research. 1994;**9**(5): 745-751

[86] Black DM, Cummings SR, Karpf DB, Cauley JA, Thompson DE, Nevitt MC, et al. Randomised trial of effect of alendronate on risk of fracture in women with existing vertebral fractures. The Lancet. 1996;**348**(9041):1535-1541

[87] Ravn P, Bidstrup M, Wasnich RD, Davis JW, McClung MR, Balske A, et al. Alendronate and estrogen–progestin in the long-term prevention of bone loss: Four-year results from the early postmenopausal intervention cohort study: A randomized, controlled trial. Annals of Internal Medicine. 1999;**131**(12):935-942

[88] McClung MR, Geusens P, Miller PD, Zippel H, Bensen WG, Roux C, et al. Effect of risedronate on the risk of hip fracture in elderly women. New England Journal of Medicine. 2001;**344**(5):333-340

[89] Miller P, Roux C, McClung M, Adami S, Eastell R, Pack S, et al. Risedronate reduces hip fractures in patients with low femoral neck bone mineral density. Arthritis and Rheumatism. 1999;**42**(S1):S287

[90] Wierna A, Ansonnaud A, Soria de González A, González Mac Donald M, Zamudio H. Osteonecrosis maxilar postextracción dentaria en pacientes bajo tratamiento con bifosfonatos: Presentación de 2 casos clínicos. Revista Círculo Argentino de Odontología. 2009;**66**(207):14-18

[91] Bisdas S, Pinho NC, Smolarz A, Sader R, Vogl T, Mack M. Bisphosphonate-induced osteonecrosis of the jaws: CT and MRI spectrum of findings in 32 patients. Clinical Radiology. 2008;**63**(1):71-77

[92] Font RG, García MM, Martínez JO. Osteochemonecrosis of the jaws due to bisphosphonate treatments. Update. Medicina Oral, Patología Oral y Cirugía Bucal. 2008;**13**(5):318-324

[93] Anguita T, Agurto J, Roa I, Laissle G. Osteonecrosis asociada al uso de bifosfonatos: A propósito de un caso clínico. Revista Médica de Chile. 2006;**134**(9):1161-1165

[94] Dicuonzo G, Vincenzi B, Santini D, Avvisati G, Rocci L, Battistoni F, et al. Fever after zoledronic acid administration is due to increase in TNF-α and IL-6. Journal of Interferon & Cytokine Research. 2003;**23**(11):649-654

[95] Khan SA, Kanis JA, Vasikaran S, Kline W, Matuszewski B, McCloskey EV, et al. Elimination and biochemical responses to intravenous alendronate in postmenopausal osteoporosis. Journal of Bone and Mineral Research. 1997;**12**(10):1700-1707

[96] Stepensky D, Kleinberg L, Hoffman A. Bone as an effect compartment. Clinical Pharmacokinetics. 2003;**42**(10):863-881

[97] Itoh A, Akagi Y, Shimomura H, Aoyama T. Interaction between bisphosphonates and mineral water: Study of oral risedronate absorption in rats. Biological and Pharmaceutical Bulletin. 2016;**39**(3):323-328

[98] Akagi Y, Sakaue T, Yoneyama E, Aoyama T. Influence of mineral water on absorption of oral alendronate in rats. Yakugaku Zasshi. 2011;**131**(5):801-807

[99] Masarachia P, Weinreb M, Balena R, Rodan G. Comparison of the distribution of 3 H-alendronate and 3 H-etidronate in rat and mouse bones. Bone. 1996;**19**(3):281-290

[100] Veldboer K, Vielhaber T, Ahrens H, Hardes J, Streitbürger A, Karst U. Determination of zoledronic acid in human urine and blood plasma using liquid chromatography/electrospray mass spectrometry. Journal of Chromatography B. 2011;**879**(22):2073-2080

[101] Allen MR. Skeletal accumulation of bisphosphonates: Implications for osteoporosis treatment. Expert Opinion on Drug Metabolism & Toxicology. 2008;**4**(11):1371-1378

[102] Muntoni E, Canaparo R, Della Pepa C, Serpe L, Casale F, Barbera S, et al. Determination of disodium clodronate in human plasma and urine using gas-chromatography–nitrogen-phosphorous detections: Validation and application in pharmacokinetic study. Journal of Chromatography B. 2004;**799**(1):133-139

[103] Han YR, Qin X. Determination of alendronate sodium by ion chromatography with refractive index detection. Journal of Chromatography A. 1996;**719**(2):345-352

[104] Huikko K, Kostiainen R. Analysis of bisphosphonates by capillary electrophoresis–electrospray ionization mass spectrometry. Journal of Chromatography A. 2000;**872**(1):289-298

[105] Xie Z, Jiang Y, Zhang D. Simple analysis of four bisphosphonates simultaneously by reverse phase liquid chromatography using n-amylamine as volatile ion-pairing agent. Journal of Chromatography A. 2006;**1104**(1):173-178

[106] Raccor BS, Sun J, Lawrence RF, Li L, Zhang H, Somerman MJ, et al. Quantitation of zoledronic acid in murine bone by liquid chromatography coupled with tandem mass spectrometry. Journal of Chromatography B. 2013;**935**:54-60

[107] Leo GC, Darrow AL. NMR-based metabolomics of urine for the atherosclerotic mouse model using apolipoprotein-E deficient mice. Magnetic Resonance in Chemistry. 2009;**47**(S1):S20–S25

[108] Zhang J, Bowers J, Liu L, Wei S, Gowda GN, Hammoud Z, et al. Esophageal cancer metabolite biomarkers detected by LC-MS and NMR methods. PLoS One. 2012;**7**(1):e30181

[109] Mallol R, Rodriguez MA, Brezmes J, Masana L, Correig X. Human serum/plasma lipoprotein analysis by NMR: Application to the study of diabetic dyslipidemia. Progress in Nuclear Magnetic Resonance Spectroscopy. 2013;**70**:1-24

[110] Kostara CE, Papathanasiou A, Psychogios N, Cung MT, Elisaf MS, Goudevenos J, et al. NMR-based lipidomic analysis of blood lipoproteins differentiates the progression of coronary heart disease. Journal of Proteome Research. 2014;**13**(5):2585-2598

[111] Bouatra S, Aziat F, Mandal R, Guo AC, Wilson MR, Knox C, et al. The human urine metabolome. PLoS One. 2013;**8**(9):e73076

[112] Beckonert O, Keun HC, Ebbels TM, Bundy J, Holmes E, Lindon JC, et al. Metabolic profiling, metabolomic and metabonomic procedures for NMR spectroscopy of urine, plasma, serum and tissue extracts. Nature Protocols. 2007;**2**(11):2692-2703

[113] Dona AC, Jiménez B, Schäfer H, Humpfer E, Spraul M, Lewis MR, et al. Precision high-throughput proton NMR spectroscopy of human urine, serum, and plasma for large-scale metabolic phenotyping. Analytical Chemistry. 2014;**86**(19):9887-9894

[114] Richards SA, & Hollerton JC. Essential Practical NMR for Organic Chemistry. John Wiley & Sons; 2010

[115] Dieterle F, Ross A, Schlotterbeck G, Senn H. Probabilistic quotient normalization as robust method to account for dilution of complex biological mixtures. Application in 1H NMR metabonomics. Analytical Chemistry. 2006;**78**(13):4281-4290

[116] Geusens P. Emerging treatments for postmenopausal osteoporosis - focus on denosumab. Clinical Interventions in Aging. 2009;**4**:241-250

[117] Fizazi K, Lipton A, Mariette X, Body JJ, Rahim Y, Gralow JR, et al. Randomized phase II trial of denosumab in patients with bone metastases from prostate cancer, breast cancer, or other neoplasms after intravenous bisphosphonates. Journal of Clinical Oncology. 2009 Apr 1;**27**(10):1564-1571

[118] Boyle WJ, Simonet WS, Lacey DL. Osteoclast differentiation and activation. Nature. 2003;**423**(6937):337-342.

[119] Baud'Huin M, Lamoureux F, Duplomb L, Rédini F, Heymann D. RANKL, RANK, osteoprotegerin: Key partners of osteoimmunology and vascular diseases. Cellular and Molecular Life Sciences. 2007;**64**(18):2334-2350

[120] Teitelbaum SL. Osteoclasts: What do they do and how do they do it? The American Journal of Pathology. 2007;**170**(2):427-435

[121] Hofbauer LC, Heufelder AE. Role of receptor activator of nuclear factor-κB ligand and osteoprotegerin in bone cell biology. Journal of Molecular Medicine. 2001;**79**(5-6):243-253

[122] Reddy GK, Mughal TI, Roodman GD. Novel approaches in the management of myeloma-related skeletal complications. Supportive Cancer Therapy. 2006;**4**(1):15-18

[123] Romas E. Clinical applications of RANK-ligand inhibition. Internal Medicine Journal. 2009;**39**(2):110-116

[124] Bekker PJ, Holloway DL, Rasmussen AS, Murphy R, Martin SW, Leese PT, et al. A single-dose placebo-controlled study of AMG 162, a fully human monoclonal antibody to RANKL, in postmenopausal women. Journal of Bone and Mineral Research. 2004;**19**(7):1059-1066

[125] Brown JP, Prince RL, Deal C, Recker RR, Kiel DP, de Gregorio LH, et al. Comparison of the effect of denosumab and alendronate on BMD and biochemical markers of bone turnover in postmenopausal women with low bone mass: A randomized, blinded, phase 3 trial. Journal of Bone and Mineral Research. 2009;**24**(1):153-161

[126] Lipton A, Steger GG, Figueroa J, Alvarado C, Solal-Celigny P, Body JJ, et al. Extended efficacy and safety of denosumab in breast cancer patients with bone metastases not receiving prior bisphosphonate therapy. Clinical Cancer Research. 2008 Oct 15;**14**(20): 6690-6696

[127] Qi W, Tang L, He A, Yao Y, Shen Z. Risk of osteonecrosis of the jaw in cancer patients receiving denosumab: A meta-analysis of seven randomized controlled trials. International Journal of Clinical Oncology. 2014;**19**(2):403-410

[128] Scagliotti GV, Hirsh V, Siena S, Henry DH, Woll PJ, Manegold C, et al. Overall survival improvement in patients with lung cancer and bone metastases treated with denosumab versus zoledronic acid: Subgroup analysis from a randomized phase 3 study. Journal of Thoracic Oncology. 2012;**7**(12):1823-1829

[129] Taylor K, Middlefell L, Mizen K. Osteonecrosis of the jaws induced by anti-RANK ligand therapy. British Journal of Oral and Maxillofacial Surgery. 2010;**48**(3):221-223

[130] Aghaloo TL, Dry SM, Mallya S, Tetradis S. Stage 0 osteonecrosis of the jaw in a patient on denosumab. Journal of Oral and Maxillofacial Surgery. 2014;**72**(4):702-716

[131] Matsushita Y, Hayashida S, Morishita K, Sakamoto H, Naruse T, Sakamoto Y, et al. Denosumab-associated osteonecrosis of the jaw affects osteoclast formation and differentiation: Pathological features of two cases. Molecular and Clinical Oncology. 2016;**4**(2):191-194

[132] Tenore G, Palaia G, Gaimari G, Brugnoletti O, Bove L, Lo Giudice R, et al. Medication-related osteonecrosis of the jaws (MRONJ): Etiological update. Senses and Sciences. 2014;**1**(10):147-152

Chapter 5

Medication-Related Osteonecrosis of the Jaw

Kenji Yamagata, Fumihiko Uchida, Naomi Kanno,
Toru Yanagawa and Hiroki Bukawa

Additional information is available at the end of the chapter

http://dx.doi.org/10.5772/67980

Abstract

Osteonecrosis of the jaw (ONJ) is a common side effect of antiresorptive drugs that are administered to cancer patients for bone metastasis, multiple myeloma, and osteoporosis. Since both bisphosphonate (BP) and denosumab show anti-bone resorption effects with ONJ, antiresorptive agent-related ONJ (ARONJ) has been suggested as a comprehensive term encompassing both BP-related osteonecrosis of the jaw (BRONJ) and denosumab-related osteonecrosis of the jaw (DRONJ). The term medication-related osteonecrosis of the jaw (MRONJ) is proposed as ARONJ with the antiangiogenic inhibitors or molecularly targeted drugs-related ONJ. Suppression of bone remodeling may contribute to the development of osteonecrosis and results in inadequate osteoclast activity to allow healing of the extraction socket. Infection is a major factor in the development of MRONJ. The major treatment goals for patients at risk of developing or who have MRONJ are prioritization and support of continued oncologic treatment in patients receiving antiresorptive and antiangiogenic therapy. To minimize the development of MRONJ in patients at risk, regular dental examinations are encouraged. Oral hygiene should be improved and local infection is managed as early as possible. The use of antibiotics before and after oral surgical procedures has been demonstrated to lower the risk of MRONJ.

Keywords: medication-related osteonecrosis of the jaw (MRONJ), bisphosphonate (BP), receptor activator nuclear factor kB ligand (RANKL) inhibitor, BP-related osteonecrosis of the jaw (BRONJ), denosumab-related osteonecrosis of the jaw (DRONJ), antiresorptive agent, antiresorptive agent-related osteonecrosis of the jaw (ARONJ), angiogenesis inhibitors

1. Introduction

Osteonecrosis of the jaw is a common side effect of antiresorptive drugs that are administered to cancer patients for bone metastasis, multiple myeloma, and osteoporosis. Antiresorptive medications contain bisphosphonates and the receptor activator nuclear factor kB ligand (RANKL) inhibitor [1].

On the other hand, denosumab, a human IGG2 monoclonal antibody against RANKL, is a therapeutic agent for bone metastasis and osteoporosis, with a half-life of approximately 1 month. Unlike bisphosphonates (BPs), which promotes apoptosis in osteoclasts, denosumab inhibits osteoclastic bone resorption without causing apoptosis. Furthermore, denosumab is not deposited in the bone and thus does not persist for long periods of time, as is the case with BPs, and so the effects of denosumab are reversible [2]. However, patients treated with denosumab also developed ONJ (denosumab-related ONJ [DRONJ]), which was clinically indistinguishable from BRONJ and occurred at almost the same rates [3].

Since both BP and denosumab which show anti-bone resorption effects through different molecular mechanisms of action are associated with ONJ, antiresorptive agent-related ONJ (ARONJ) has been suggested as a comprehensive term encompassing both BRONJ and DRONJ [4]. The American Association of Oral and Maxillofacial Surgeons (AAOMS) has proposed the term "medication-related osteonecrosis of the jaw" (MRONJ), based on observations that antiangiogenic inhibitors and molecularly targeted drugs such as tyrosine kinase inhibitors are also infrequently associated with ONJ or increase the incidence of BRONJ/DRONJ in cancer patients receiving BPs or denosumab, although global consensus has not yet been established [5].

The number of patients with MRONJ has grown recently. Medication-related osteonecrosis of the jaw (MRONJ) is defined as exposed bone in the oral cavity or extra-oral fistula in the maxillofacial region for more than 8 weekswith the treatment of antiresorptive or antiangiogenic agents for more than 8 weeks. These patients have no history of radiotherapy or metastatic disease in the jaw. We present about the details, pathophysiology, diagnosis, staging and treatment, risk factor, and prevention of MRONJ in below paragraphs in this chapter.

2. Antiresorptive and antiangiogenic medications

2.1. Bisphosphonates (BPs)

Intravenous BPs are antiresorptive agents and administered for cancer–related conditions; hypercalcemia of malignancy, skeletal-related events (SREs) associated with bone metastases in the context of solid tumors (for example breast, prostate and lung cancers), and lytic lesions of multiple myeloma. These medications have a significant positive effect for the quality of life of patients with bone metastatic cancer [5]. Oral BPs are approved for the treatment of osteoporosis and osteopenia. They have been used in less common conditions, such as paget disease of bone and osteogenesis imperfection. The most common use is for osteopenia and osteoporosis [6].

2.2. RANKL inhibitor (denosumab)

The receptor activator of RANKL inhibitor (denosumab) inhibits osteoclast function and bone resorption. There is a decrease in the risk of vertebral, nonvertebral, and hip fractures in osteoporotic patients for administrating denosumab subcutaneously every 6 months. Moreover, monthly administration of denosumab is effective for decreasing SREs-related metastatic bone disease from solid tumors [7, 8]. In contrast to BPs, denosumab do not bind to bone and their effects of bone remodeling continue within 6 months [5].

2.3. Antiangiogenic medications

Angiogenesis inhibitors interfere with the formation of new blood vessels by connecting to many signaling molecules and disrupting the angiogenesis-signaling cascade. These medications are administered for gastrointestinal tumors, renal cell carcinoma, neuroendocrine tumors, and other malignancies [5].

3. Pathophysiology

The pathophysiology of MRONJ is well unknown and considered to be multifactorial. Suppressed bone remodeling may contribute to the development of osteonecrosis, and in inadequate osteoclast activity disturbed cure the extraction socket. Infection is a major factor for the development of MRONJ. Bacteria stimulate bone resorption and contribute to bone necrosis [9].

3.1. Incidence of MRONJ

The reported incidence of MRONJ varies by study, and there are no reliable epidemiological data derived from evidenced-based medicine. This chapter follows the data cited by the International Task Force on ONJ [10].

3.1.1. Patients with osteoporosis

1. BRONJ

   The incidence is 1.04–69/100,000 patients per year treated with orally administered BPs and 0–90/100,000 patients per year treated with intravenous administration. The incidence of ONJ in patients with osteoporosis treated with oral/intravenous nitrogen-containing BPs ranges from 0.001 to 0.01%, which is estimated to be almost the same or slightly higher than the incidence (0.01%) of ONJ in the general population [10].

2. DRONJ

   The incidence is 0–30.2/100,000 patients per year [10].

3.1.2. Cancer patients

The incidence of ONJ in cancer patients is higher than that in patients with osteoporosis. Prospective studies on the incidence of ONJ were conducted in cancer patients treated with zoledronic acid or denosumab. Among 5723 patients with breast, prostate, and other solid cancer and multiple myeloma, there were 89 ONJ cases in total, 52 in the denosumab, and 37 in the zoledronic acid-treated. The incidence in the denosumab-treated was 1.8% and 1.3% in the zoledronic acid [3, 11].

3.2. Uniqueness of the jaw bone [12]

There are several unique anatomical and microbiological characteristics of the jaw bone, which could be responsible for the specific occurrence of MRONJ. These characteristics are not found in bones or in other parts of the body.

The teeth erupt from the jawbone, breaking the oral epithelium, allowing infectious factors, agents, and microbes in the oral cavity to directly invade the jaw bone through the gap between the epithelium and the teeth or via root canal.

1. The oral mucosa covering the jawbone is thin, and infection caused by mucosal injury spreads to the jawbone beneath the mucosa.
2. More than 800 types of resident bacteria (10^{11} to 10^{12} cm^{-3}) inhabit dental plaque and can serve as a source of infection in the oral cavity.
3. Inflammation due to tooth decay, pulpitis, periapical lesions, or periodontal disease extends to the jawbone.
4. The jawbone is exposed to the oral cavity following invasive dental treatments including tooth extraction, leading to infection.

3.3. Suppression of bone turnover

BPs and denosumab inhibit osteoclast differentiation and function, increased apoptosis, and decreased bone resorption and remodeling [2, 13, 14]. Osteoclast differentiation and function act as an effective role for bone remodeling for skeletal sites, but MRONJ occurs only primarily within the alveolar bone of jaw [15]. An increased remodeling rate in the jaw may be considered for the differential predisposition of MRONJ to occur in the jaws compared with other bones in the axial or appendicular skeleton [5].

The relation between excessive suppression of C-terminal telopeptides of type I collagen (CTX), a bone resorption marker, and MRONJ incidence has been reported in several studies. However, a correlation between CTX level and severity of MRONJ has not been observed. There is still much controversy on whether a relationship exists between CTX levels and MRONJ incidence [16–18].

3.4. Infection/inflammation

The risk factors have been implicated dental disease or bacterial infection in MRONJ. Although dental extraction was performed in most reported cases of MRONJ, these teeth commonly contracted with periodontal or periapical diseases. Inflammation or infection has long been considered an important component of MRONJ [19, 20].

3.5. Angiogenesis inhibition

Angiogenesis is a process that involves growth, migration, and differentiation of endothelial cells to form new blood vessels. Angiogenesis favorably influences tumor growth and influences tumor invasion of vessels, resulting in tumor metastasis. Osteonecrosis is classically considered as an interruption in vascular supply or avascular necrosis; therefore, it is not surprising that inhibition of angiogenesis is a leading hypothesis in MRONJ pathophysiology [21, 22].

3.6. Soft tissue toxicity

Although BPs primarily targets the osteoclast and bind to hydroxyapatite in bone, soft tissue toxicity has been reported. In contrast to BPs, no soft tissue toxicity has been reported with denosumab [23].

4. Diagnosis of MRONJ [5, 12]

MRONJ is definitively diagnosed when the following three conditions are met:

1. Patients have a history of treatment with BP, denosumab, and antiangiogenic agents.
2. Patients have no history of radiation therapy to the jaw. Bone lesions of MRONJ must be differentiated from cancer metastasis to the jawbone by histological examination.
3. Exposure of alveolar bone in the oral cavity, jaw, and/or face is continuously observed for longer than 8 weeks after first detection by a medical or dental expert, or the bone is palpable in the intra- or extra-oral fistula for longer than 8 weeks.

5. Staging of MRONJ

The clinical manifestations and staging of MRONJ are summarized in **Table 1**. Paresthesia of the chin, including the lower lip (Vincent's symptom), in patients treated with BP is an early sign of MRONJ, before alveolar bone exposure is detected [5, 12].

1. At risk

   There is no apparent necrotic bone in asymptomatic patients who have been treated with intravenous or oral antiresorptive or antiangiogenic therapy.

	Staging of MRONJ	Treatment strategies
At risk	No apparent necrotic bone in patients who have been treated with oral or intravenous bisphosphonates	No treatment indicated and patient education
Stage 0	No clinical evidence of necrotic bone but nonspecific clinical findings, radiographic changes, and symptoms	Systemic management, including use of pain medication and antibiotics
Stage 1	Exposed and necrotic bone or fistula that probes to bone in patients who are asymptomatic and have no evidence of infection	Antibiotic mouth rinse, clinical follow-up on a quarterly basis, patient education, and review of indications for continued bisphosphonate therapy
Stage 2	Exposed and necrotic bone or fistula that probes to bone associated with infection as evidenced by pain and erythema in the region of exposed bone with or without purulent drainage	Symptomatic treatment with oral antibiotics, oral bacterial mouth rinse, pain control, debridement to relieve soft tissue irritation, and infection control
Stage 3	Exposed and necrotic bone or a fistula that probes to bone in patients with pain, infection, and >1 of the following: exposed and necrotic bone extending beyond the region of alveolar bone (i.e., inferior border and ramus in mandible, maxillary sinus, and zygoma in maxilla) resulting in pathologic fracture, extra-oral fistula, oral antral or oral nasal communication, or osteolysis extending to inferior border of the mandible or sinus floor	Antibacterial mouth rinse, antibiotic therapy and pain control, surgical debridement or resection for longer-term palliation of infection and pain

Table 1. Staging and treatment strategies.

2. Stage 0 (unexposed bone variant)

These patients have no clinical evidence of necrotic bone, but nonspecific clinical findings, radiographic changes, and symptoms.

3. Stage 1

Stage 1 is defined as asymptomatic exposed and necrotic bone or a fistula that probes to bone. These patients have no evidence of infection and may present with radiographic findings localized to the alveolar bone region.

4. Stage 2 (**Figures 1–4**)

Stage 2 is defined as exposed and necrotic bone or a fistula that probes to bone with evidence of infection. These patients are typically symptomatic. These patients also may present with radiographic findings which are localized to the alveolar bone region.

5. Stage 3 (**Figures 5–11**)

Stage 3 is defined as exposed and necrotic bone or fistula that probes to bone with evidence of infection and at least one of the following:

(i) Exposed necrotic bone extending beyond the region of alveolar bone to the inferior border and ramus in the mandible, maxillary sinus, and zygoma in the maxilla.

(ii) Pathologic fracture.

(iii) Extra-oral fistula.

(iv) Oral antral or oral nasal communication.

(v) Osteolysis extending to the inferior border of the mandible or sinus floor.

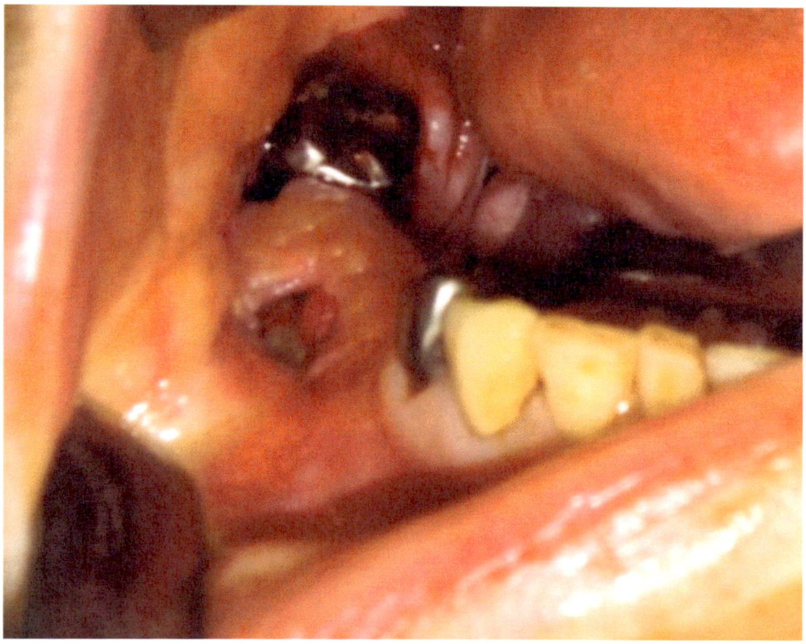

Figure 1. MRONJ (Stage 2). Intraoral examination. The necrotic bone with evidence of infection is exposed. The permission to use the picture of this figure from the Ishiyaku Publisher, Inc. in Japan.

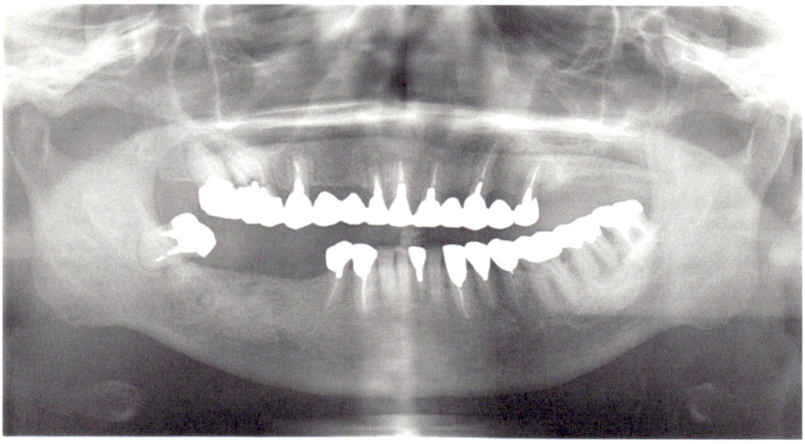

Figure 2. Panoramic X-ray. The permission to use the picture of this figure from the Ishiyaku Publisher, Inc. in Japan.

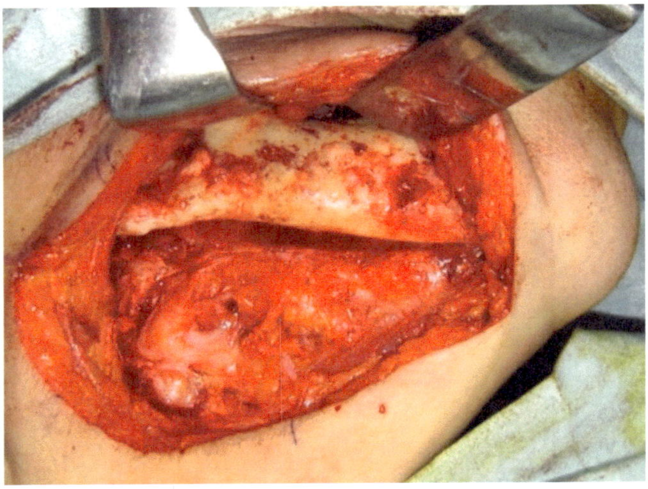

Figure 3. The segmental resection of the mandible is performed under general anesthesia. There is partial bone defect. The permission to use the picture of this figure from the Ishiyaku Publisher, Inc. in Japan.

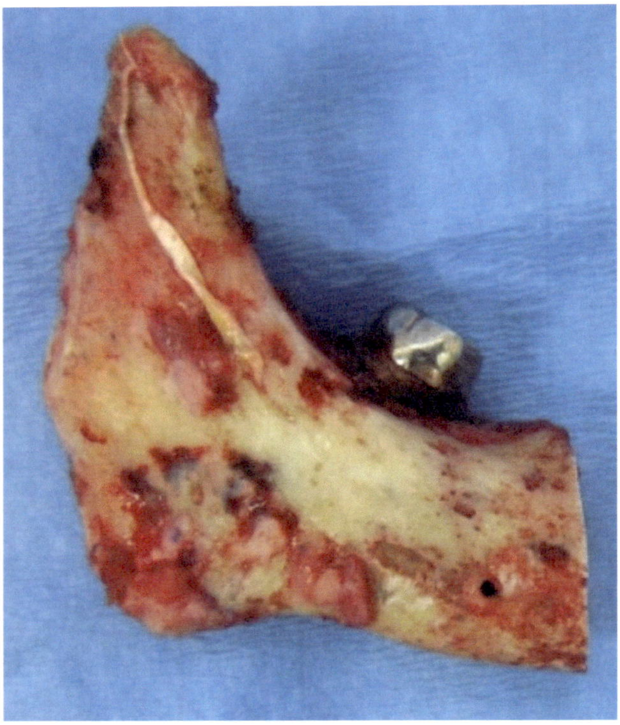

Figure 4. The resected specimen of the mandible. The permission to use the picture of this figure from the Ishiyaku Publisher, Inc. in Japan.

http://dx.doi.org/10.5772/67980

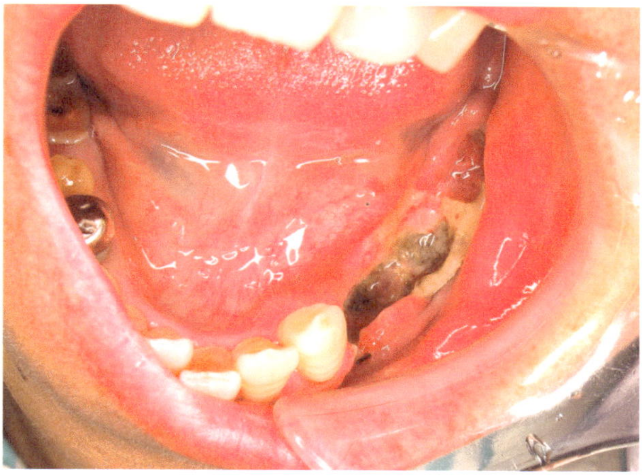

Figure 5. MRONJ (Stage 3). Intraoral examination. The necrotic bone with evidence of infection is exposed. The molar teeth are lost naturally. The permission to use the pictures of this figure from the Ishiyaku Publisher, Inc. in Japan.

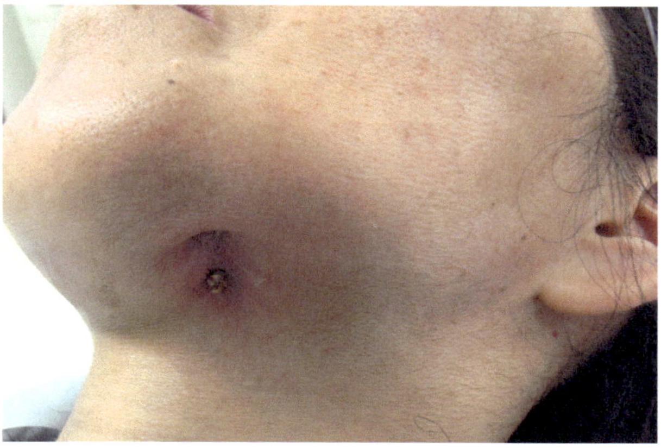

Figure 6. Necrotic bone extending beyond the region of alveolar bone is exposed, and extra-oral fistula is appeared. The permission to use the picture of this figure from the Ishiyaku Publisher, Inc. in Japan.

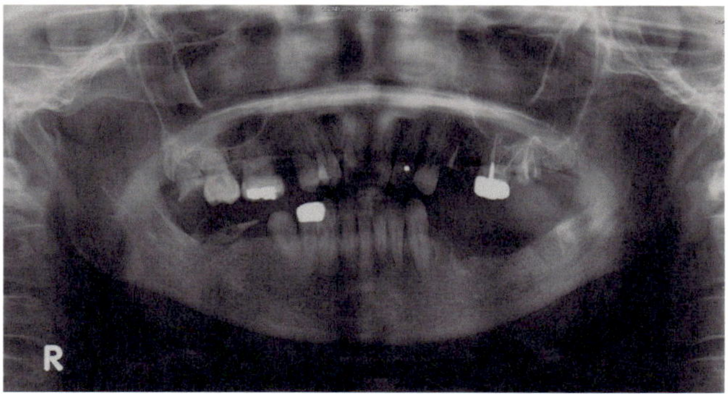

Figure 7. The panoramic X-ray. Regions of osteosclerosis involving the alveolar bone of lost molar teeth are depicted. The permission to use the picture of this figure from the Ishiyaku Publisher, Inc. in Japan.

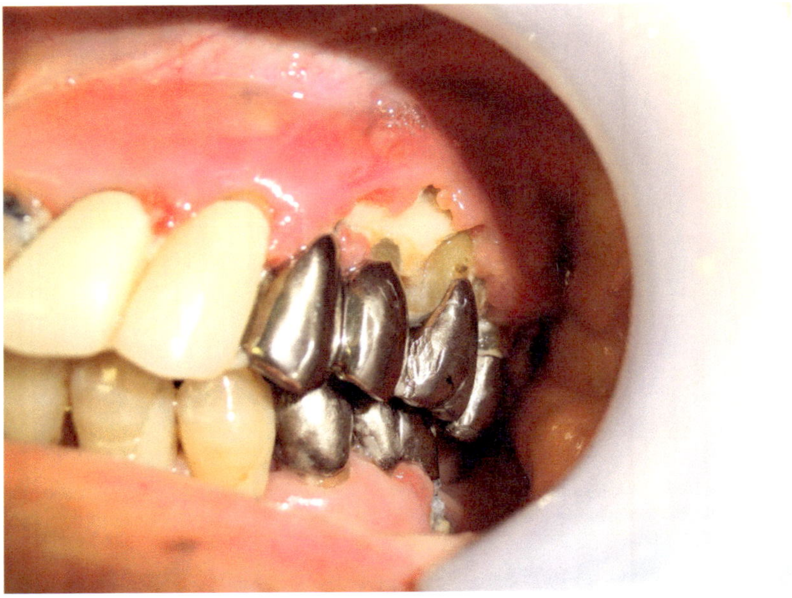

Figure 8. MRONJ (Stage 3). Sequester is extended to maxillary sinus. Oral antral communication is made. The permission to use the picture of this figure from the Ishiyaku Publisher, Inc. in Japan.

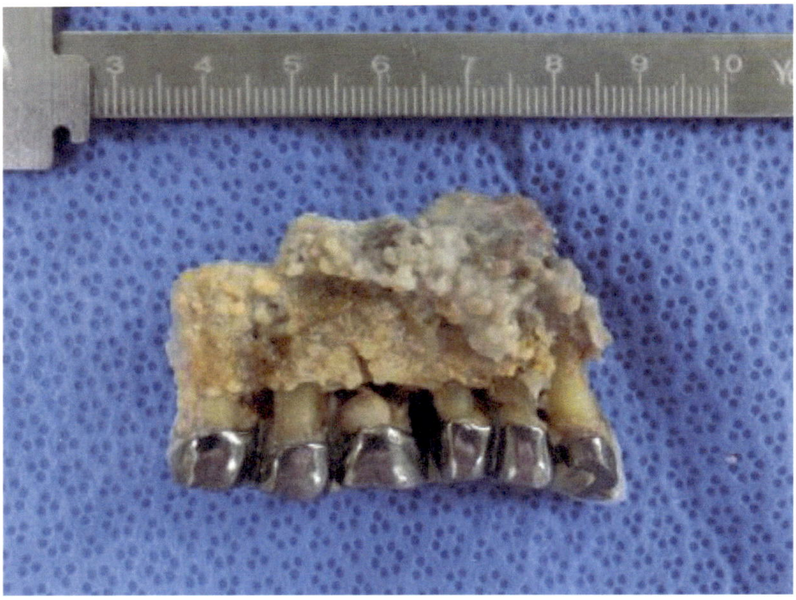

Figure 9. The sequester and six teethes are removed under local anesthesia. The oral antral communication is made at the anterior part of defect. The permission to use the picture of this figure from the Ishiyaku Publisher, Inc. in Japan.

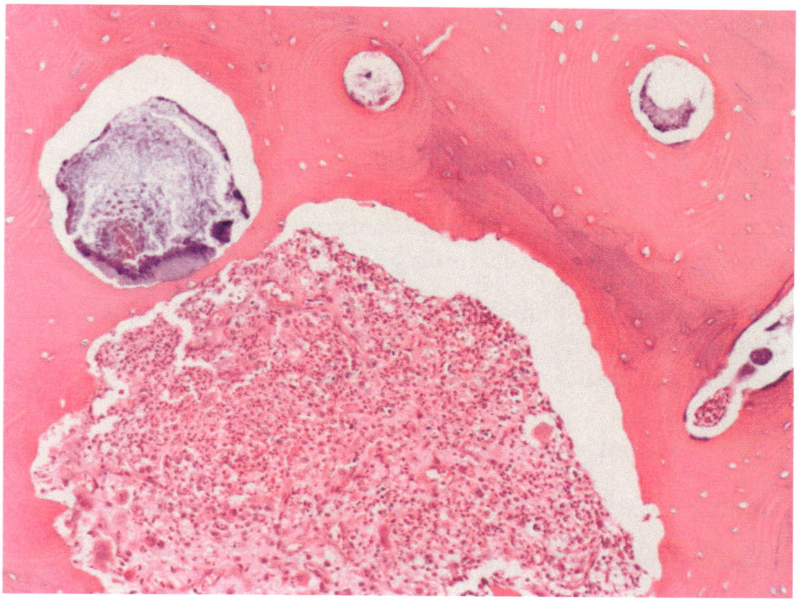

Figure 10. The necrotic bone and infiltrating inflammatory cells. The stimulating micrograms are observed (HE staining: 100×). The permission to use the picture of this figure from the Ishiyaku Publisher, Inc. in Japan.

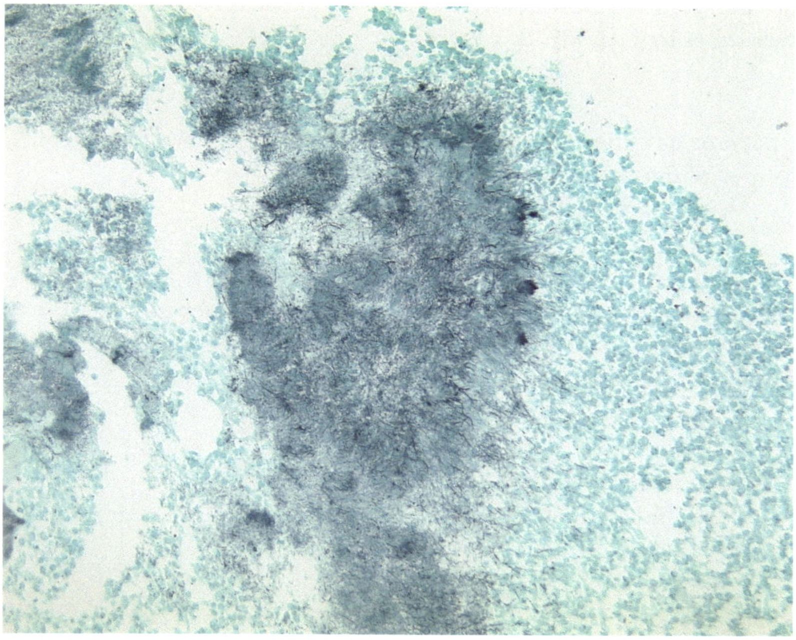

Figure 11. Actinomycetes stained with Grocott in the granulation tissue (Grocott staining). The permission to use the picture of this figure from the Ishiyaku Publisher, Inc. in Japan.

6. Treatment strategies for MRONJ

6.1. Treatment goals

The treatment goals for patients at risk of developing or who have MRONJ are prioritization and support of continued cancer treatment in patients receiving intra venous antiresorptive and antiangiogenic therapy [5, 12]. Cancer patients can benefit greatly from the therapeutic effect from antiresorptive agents by controlling SREs.

Maintenance of patient quality of life (QOL) is done by relieving symptoms, including pain, pus discharge, and paresthesia, and by control of infection. Moreover, patient education and routine follow-up for oral health care are needed by dental expert.

6.2. Stage-specific treatment strategies

Therapeutic strategies based on MRONJ stages are summarized in **Table 1** [5].

Treatment of MRONJ varies with the stages of the disease. However, regardless of the stage, the protocol must include treating dental and periodontal diseases, maintaining and improving oral health with antibacterial mouthwash, and systemically administering antibacterial agents. To ensure success with surgical treatment, the complete elimination of MRONJ lesions and closure of surgical wounds is critical, along with systemic administration of antibacterial agents. For patients with a history of malignant tumors, histopathological examination of all necrotic bones removed will be needed to exclude the possibility that excised MRONJ lesions are tumor metastases to the jaw [12].

1. At risk

   These patients have no exposed bone and requirement of any treatment. They should be informed of the risks of developing to MRONJ.

2. Stage 0

   These patients receive the treatment of symptomatic disease and conservative management of caries and periodontal disease. Systemic management, including use of pain medication and antibiotics are indicated. These patients should be prevented of progression to a higher stage.

3. Stage 1

   These patients are indicated with medical management of the use for oral antimicrobial rinses, such as chlorhexidine 0.12%. No immediate surgery is required.

4. Stage 2

   These patients are indicated with oral antimicrobial rinses in combination with administrating antibiotic therapy. The debridement to relieve soft tissue irritation and infection control is needed.

http://dx.doi.org/10.5772/67980

5. Stage 3

    These patients are benefit from debridement, including resection, in combination with antibiotic therapy. Symptomatic patients with stage 3 may require resection and immediate reconstruction with reconstruction plate or an obturator.

Regardless of the disease stage, mobile bony sequestra should be removed to facilitate soft tissue healing. The extraction of symptomatic teeth within exposed necrotic bone should be considered because it is unlikely that the extraction will exacerbate the established necrotic process.

6.3. Treatment with parathyroid hormone (teriparatide)

Systemic administration of low doses of recombinant parathyroid hormone (teriparatide) has been shown to resolve ONJ symptoms and promote a cure. Japanese studies have also shown improved bone regeneration and healing in ONJ lesions with the use of teriparatide [24, 25]. It should also be noted that administration of teriparatide is contraindicated in patients with metastatic bone tumors, and its total dose and period of administration are restricted as well.

7. Risk factors for MRONJ

Proposed risk factors for MRONJ are listed in **Table 2** [12]. Among these factors, invasive dental treatments, such as tooth extraction, dental implant, or apical/periodontal surgery, are definitive local risk factors for MRONJ.

7.1. Dental implants and MRONJ [12]

Recent reports suggested that dental implant procedures performed in patients with cancer or osteoporosis prior to treatment with BPs are not likely associated with subsequent occurrence of MRONJ, if oral health is appropriately managed. However, dental implant performed during or after BP treatment is a potential risk factor for MRONJ [26, 27].

It is unknown whether dental implant is a risk factor in patients receiving denosumab. Implants are not advised for cancer patients who are receiving antiresorptive treatment, and alternative dental measures are recommended. On the other hand, in patients with osteoporosis, dental implant may be performed in cases in which physicians and dentists agree that dental implants are essential for improving the systemic and oral health of patients [12].

7.2. Coadministered agents and MRONJ

Antiangiogenic agents and tyrosine kinase inhibitors, which are essentially administered as adjuvants in the treatment of cancer patients, have been shown to cause MRONJ, albeit very rarely, when used alone, or to increase the incidence of MRONJ when used concomitantly with BP or denosumab [28].

1. Local
Invasive dental treatments including bone (e.g., tooth extraction, dental implants, apical/periodontal surgery)
Ill-fitting dentures and excessive bite force
Poor sanitation in the oral cavity, periodontal disease, and gingival abscess inflammatory disease, including apical periodontitis
Common site: mandible > maxilla, mandibular torus, palatal torus, and mylohyoid line torus
Root canal and orthodontic treatments are not considered to be risk factors
2. Antiresorptive agents
Nitrogen-containing bisphosphonates (BPs) > nonnitrogen-containing BPs
Denosumab
Drugs for malignant tumor > drug for osteoporosis
Drug for malignant tumor (Zometa, Aredia, Teiroc, Ranmark)
Drug for osteoporosis (Didronel, Fosamac, Bonalon, Actonel, Benet, Bonoteo, Recalbon, Bonbiba and Pralia)
Dose and administration period
3. Systemic
Cancer (breast, prostate, lung, renal and colon cancer, multiple myeloma, and other cancers)
Diabetes, rheumatoid arthritis, hypocalcemia, hypoparathyroidism, osteomalacia, vitamin D deficiency, renal dialysis, anemia, and Paget's disease of bone
4. Congenital
Single-nucleotide polymorphisms (SNPs) in MMP-2 and cytochrome P450-2C genes
5. Lifestyle
Smoking, drinking alcohol, and obesity
6. Coadministered agents
Anticancer agents, corticosteroid, and erythropoietin
Angiogenic inhibitors (e.g., thalidomide, sunitinib, and lenalidomide)
Tyrosine kinase inhibitors

Table 2. Risk factors for MRONJ.

8. Prevention of MRONJ

To minimize the development of ONJ in patients at risk, regular dental examinations are encouraged. Oral hygiene should be improved and local infection is managed as early as possible. The use of antibiotics before and after oral surgical procedures has been demonstrated to lower the risk of ONJ [29, 30]. Antimicrobial mouth rinses may also be useful in lowering the risk of ONJ [30, 31].

All necessary oral surgeries in oncology patients should ideally be completed before the initiation of high-dose antiresorptive therapy. For oncology patient requiring high-dose intravenous BPs or high-dose denosumab, dental radiographs should be completed before medication begins. Any invasive dental procedure including dental extractions or implants should ideally be completed before the initiation of antiresorptive therapy. Nonurgent procedures should be delayed if necessary. If ONJ develops, it is recommended that the antiresorptive drug therapy should be withheld until soft tissue closure with a well-epithelialized mucosa is achieved [32].

There is currently no evidence that interruption of drug therapy in patients requiring dental procedures reduces the risk of ONJ or the progression of the disease [29]. (BPs) that have long-term skeletal retention and cessation for weeks or months may not impact remodeling significantly. However, BPs do have increased skeletal uptake at the sites of local bone injury, and withholding BP therapy following oral surgery may be of use in reducing the local deposition in the mandible and maxilla after oral surgery. In individuals with significant risk factors for ONJ, including oncology patients on high-dose antiresorptive therapy as well as those individuals with multiple risk factors for ONJ, it may be of benefit to withhold BP or denosumab therapy following oral surgery until soft tissue healing occurs [32].

In determining the suitability if drug interruption, it is necessary to weigh the risks of ONJ with the risk of skeletal-related events in oncology patients and the risk of fracture in those with osteoporosis. The decision to hold therapy should be jointly made between the oral surgeon and the physician treating the underlying osteoporosis. Patients with osteoporosis receiving BP or denosumab may continue with therapy if a dental procedure including extraction and implant surgery is required [4]. The decision to continue or hold antiresorptive therapy should be made by the dental health provider in consultation with the patient's physician [32].

8.1. Dental treatments and discontinuation of antiresorptive therapy

8.1.1. Dental treatments in patients who are to receive antiresorptive therapy

Before initiation of antiresorptive therapy, it is wise to request that patients visit a dentist for control of oral health to prevent the occurrence of ONJ. Ideally, all dental treatments should be completed 2 weeks before starting antiresorptive treatment. However, in the event that antiresorptive treatment cannot be delayed due to progression of bone metastases or high risk of fracture, administration of antiresorptive agents in parallel with dental treatments may be acceptable. During antiresorptive treatment, patients should be instructed by physicians to adhere to routine dental visits for oral examination [12].

8.1.2. Dental treatments in patients receiving antiresorptive agents

1. Discontinuation of BPs before starting dental treatment

There is a considerable controversy around the question of whether discontinuation (drug holiday) of BPs for a certain period of time before invasive dental treatment is effective in preventing or reducing occurrence of BRONJ. A BP drug holiday before starting invasive dental treatment is not logically supported from background information [12]. The American Association of Oral and Maxillofacial (AAOMS) and other groups have described an increased incidence of BRONJ who were treated with BPs for longer than 4 years. From these results, AAOMS recommended that, for patients receiving antiresorptive therapy for longer than 4 years and who have low fracture risk but potentially high risk for BRONJ, discontinuation of antiresorptive treatment for approximately 2 months before invasive dental treatment should be considered, in consultation with the physician [5]. Thus, no consensus has yet been reached regarding whether a BP drug holiday before invasive dental treatment is appropriate and necessary for prevention of BRONJ [12].

2. Suggested dental treatment in patients with cancer and osteoporosis who are receiving BPs

   Dental experts will need to educate patients on the importance of daily oral sanitation, including how to clean the oral cavity after each meal and rinse their mouths with antibacterial mouthwash. Subsequently, dentists begin conservative dental treatment without discontinuation of BPs. In the case that invasive dental treatment such as removal of the teeth responsible for BRONJ is inevitable, however, antibacterial agents will be administered to the patients in advance, and invasive dental treatments should be restricted to the minimum extent and area possible to avoid discontinuation of BP treatment [12].

3. Suggested dental treatment in patients with cancer and osteoporosis who are receiving denosumab

   For cancer patients with bone metastases, studies have found that the benefits of denosumab are highly superior to those of zoledronic acid [11]. The incidence of DRONJ and BRONJ, however, was found to be similar in patients with cancer [3]. Similar to case of patients treated with BPs, dentists perform conservative dental treatment without drug holiday. Invasive dental treatments, if inevitable, can be conducted without a drug holiday following appropriate infection control. Given that denosumab is administered to osteoporotic patients once every 6 months and the half-life of denosumab is approximately 1 month, there is an ample window of time within the 6-month interval to plan for dental treatments [12].

4. Discontinuation of antiresorptive therapy after invasive dental treatment

   Antiresorptive agents may interfere with the healing of surgical wounds, especially epithelialization [33]. The decision to continue or discontinue antiresorptive treatment must be made jointly by the physician and dentist based on fracture risk, and the status of healing of surgical wounds in the oral cavity.

5. Timing of resumption of antiresorptive therapy

   The time at which to resume antiresorptive administration after a drug holiday is dependent on the balance between the healing of surgical wounds and control of the primary disease. If fracture risk or bone metastasis is well-controlled, resumption of antiresorptive treatment is recommended approximately 2 months after invasive dental procedure, when the damaged alveolar bones are expected to have healed. However, if fracture risk is high or bone metastasis progresses during the drug holiday and resumption of antiresorptive therapy is urgent, it may resume antiresorptive drug with no sign of infection around surgical wounds and epithelialization of the surgical site at 2 weeks after invasive dental treatment, when epithelialization of the surgical site is almost complete, may be the earliest possibility [12].

http://dx.doi.org/10.5772/67980

9. Case report of the patient of brain abscesses caused by MRONJ [34]

Reports of brain abscesses caused by MRONJ are very rare. The case of a 76-year-old man with terminal-stage prostatic carcinoma and a brain abscess caused by MRONJ at the maxilla with conscious loss is presented here. The zoledronic acid and denosumab were administered for bone metastasis. In the case of maxillary, MRONJ spreads beyond the maxillary sinus into the ethmoid sinus and into the brain. For the brain abscess, an antibiotic regimen based on ceftriaxone and metronidazole and a sequestrectomy contributed to a successful outcome (**Figures 12–15**).

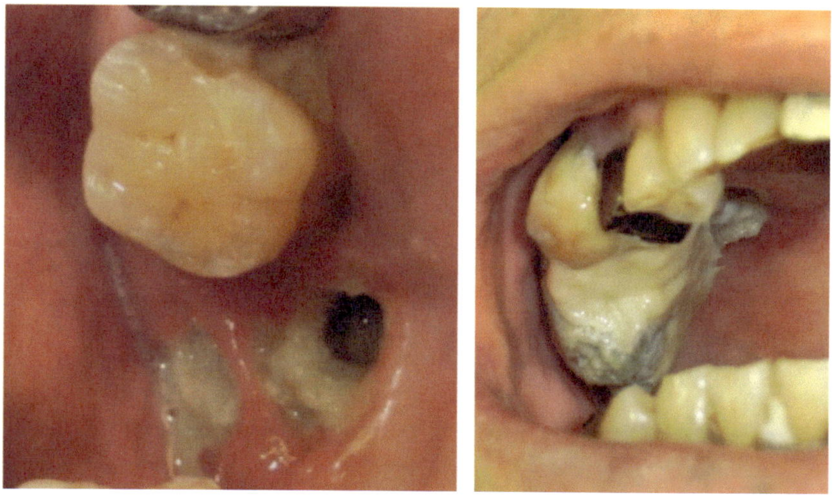

Figure 12. Intra-oral examination. The 17 was lost naturally 2 months from the first visit and sequester was revealed. The sequester expanded in 8 months from socket.

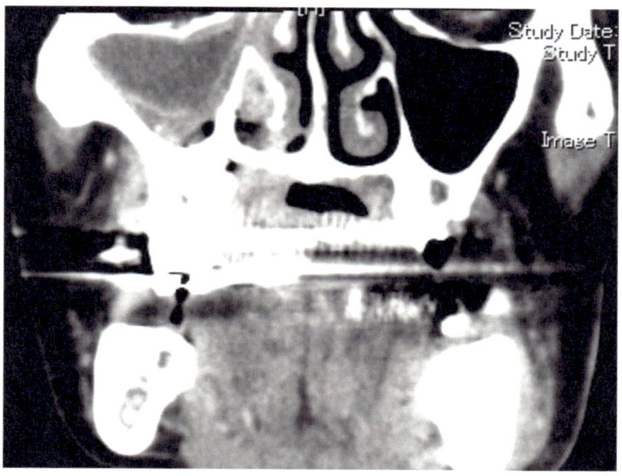

Figure 13. Preoperative CT. Abscess formation is revealed in right maxillary sinus.

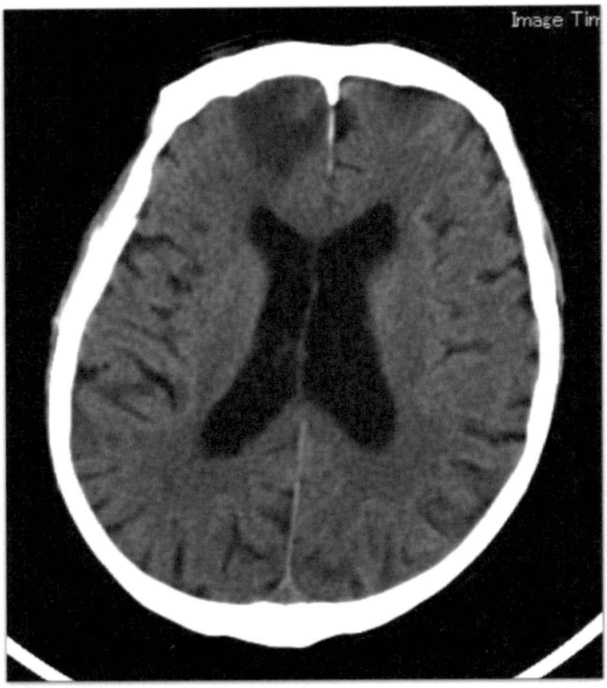

Figure 14. CT after conscious lost in ER. The absorption image in right frontal lobe is revealed.

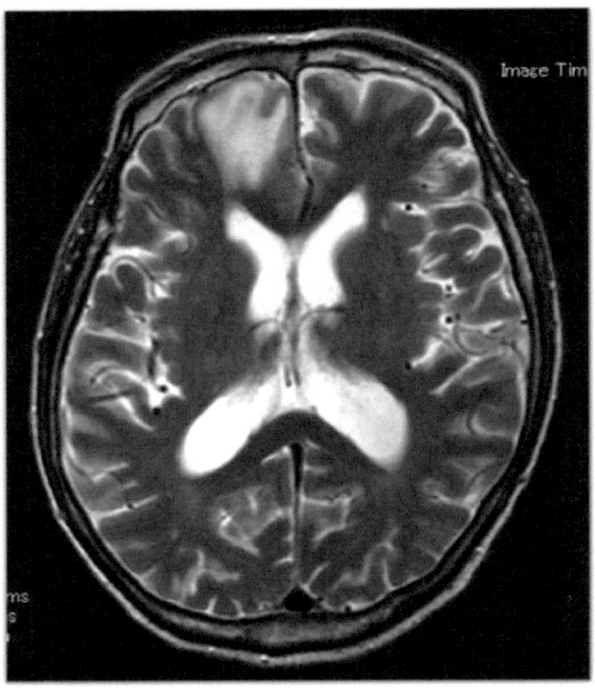

Figure 15. MRI (T2WI) after conscious lost in ER. Right frontal lobe abscess is depicted.

10. Conclusion

Medication-related osteonecrosis of the jaw (MRONJ) is a common side effect of antiresorptive drugs, which are administered to cancer patients for bone metastasis, multiple myeloma, and osteoporosis. All necessary oral surgeries in oncology patients should ideally be completed before the initiation of high-dose antiresorptive therapy, and to minimize the development of ONJ in patients at risk, regular dental examinations are encouraged. Oral hygiene should be improved and local infection should be managed as early as possible.

Author details

Kenji Yamagata*, Fumihiko Uchida, Naomi Kanno, Toru Yanagawa and Hiroki Bukawa

*Address all correspondence to: y-kenji@md.tsukuba.ac.jp

Department of Oral and Maxillofacial Surgery, Faculty of Medicine, University of Tsukuba, Tsukuba, Japan

References

[1] Marx RE. Pamidronate (Aredia) and zoledronate (Zometa) induced avascular necrosis of the jaws: a growing epidemic. J Oral Maxillofac Surg. 2003;**61**(9):1115-7.

[2] Baron R, Ferrari S, Russell RGG. Denosumab and bisphosphonates: different mechanisms of action and effects. Bone. 2011;**48**(4):677-92.

[3] Saad F, Brown JE, Van Poznak C, Ibrahim T, Stemmer SM, Stopeck AT, et al. Incidence, risk factors, and outcomes of osteonecrosis of the jaw: integrated analysis from three blinded active-controlled phase III trials in cancer patients with bone metastases. Ann Oncol. 2012;**23**(5):1341-7.

[4] Hellstein JW, Adler RA, Edwards B, Jacobsen PL, Kalmar JR, Koka S, et al. Managing the care of patients receiving antiresorptive therapy for prevention and treatment of osteoporosis: executive summary of recommendations from the American dental association council on scientific affairs. J Am Dent Assoc. 2011;**142**(11):1243-51.

[5] Ruggiero SL, Dodson TB, Fantasia J, Goodday R, Aghaloo T, Mehrotra B, et al. American association of oral and maxillofacial surgeons position paper on medication-related osteonecrosis of the jaw—2014 update. J Oral Maxillofac Surg. 2014;**72**(10):1938-56.

[6] Delmas PD. The use of bisphosphonates in the treatment of osteoporosis. Curr Opin Rheumatol. 2005;**17**(4):462-6.

[7] Cummings SR, San Martin J, McClung MR, Siris ES, Eastell R, Reid IR, et al. Denosumab for prevention of fractures in postmenopausal women with osteoporosis. N Engl J Med. 2009;**361**(8):756-65.

[8] Papapoulos S, Chapurlat R, Libanati C, Brandi ML, Brown JP, Czerwiński E, et al. Five years of denosumab exposure in women with postmenopausal osteoporosis: results from the first two years of the FREEDOM extension. J Bone Miner Res. 2012;**27**(3):694-701.

[9] Hinson AM, Smith CW, Siegel ER, Stack BC. Is bisphosphonate-related osteonecrosis of the jaw an infection? A histological and microbiological ten-year summary. Int J Dent. 2014;**2014**:452-737.

[10] Khan AA, Morrison A, Hanley DA, Felsenberg D, McCauley LK, O'Ryan F, et al. Diagnosis and management of osteonecrosis of the jaw: a systematic review and international consensus. J Bone Miner Res. 2015;**30**(1):3-23.

[11] Lipton A, Fizazi K, Stopeck AT, Henry DH, Brown JE, Yardley DA, et al. Superiority of denosumab to zoledronic acid for prevention of skeletal-related events: a combined analysis of 3 pivotal, randomised, phase 3 trials. Eur J Cancer. 2012;**48**(16):3082-92.

[12] Japanese Allied Committee on Osteonecrosis of the Jaw T, Yoneda T, Hagino H, Sugimoto T, Ohta H, Takahashi S, et al. Antiresorptive agent-related osteonecrosis of the jaw: position paper 2017 of the Japanese allied committee on osteonecrosis of the jaw. J Bone Miner Metab. 2017; **35**(1): 6-19.

[13] Russell RGG, Watts NB, Ebetino FH, Rogers MJ. Mechanisms of action of bisphosphonates: similarities and differences and their potential influence on clinical efficacy. Osteoporos Int. 2008;**19**(6):733-59.

[14] Lacey DL, Boyle WJ, Simonet WS, Kostenuik PJ, Dougall WC, Sullivan JK, et al. Bench to bedside: elucidation of the OPG-RANK-RANKL pathway and the development of denosumab. Nat Rev Drug Discov. 2012;**11**(5):401-19.

[15] Aghaloo TL, Kang B, Sung EC, Shoff M, Ronconi M, Gotcher JE, et al. Periodontal disease and bisphosphonates induce osteonecrosis of the jaws in the rat. J Bone Miner Res. 2011;**26**(8):1871-82.

[16] Kwon Y-D, Ohe J-Y, Kim D-Y, Chung D-J, Park Y-D. Retrospective study of two biochemical markers for the risk assessment of oral bisphosphonate-related osteonecrosis of the jaws: can they be utilized as risk markers? Clin Oral Implants Res. 2011;**22**(1):100-5.

[17] Kwon Y-D, Kim D-Y, Ohe J-Y, Yoo J-Y, Walter C. Correlation between serum C-terminal cross-linking telopeptide of type I collagen and staging of oral bisphosphonate-related osteonecrosis of the jaws. J Oral Maxillofac Surg. 2009;**67**(12):2644-8.

[18] Bagan J V., Jiménez Y, Gómez D, Sirera R, Poveda R, Scully C. Collagen telopeptide (serum CTX) and its relationship with the size and number of lesions in osteonecrosis of the jaws in cancer patients on intravenous bisphosphonates. Oral Oncol. 2008;**44**(11):1088-9.

[19] Ripamonti CI, Maniezzo M, Campa T, Fagnoni E, Brunelli C, Saibene G, et al. Decreased occurrence of osteonecrosis of the jaw after implementation of dental preventive measures

in solid tumour patients with bone metastases treated with bisphosphonates. The experience of the National Cancer Institute of Milan. Ann Oncol Off J Eur Soc Med Oncol. 2009;**20**(1):137-45.

[20] Dimopoulos MA, Kastritis E, Bamia C, Melakopoulos I, Gika D, Roussou M, et al. Reduction of osteonecrosis of the jaw (ONJ) after implementation of preventive measures in patients with multiple myeloma treated with zoledronic acid. Ann Oncol. 2008;**20**(1):117-20.

[21] Yamashita J, McCauley LK. Antiresorptives and osteonecrosis of the jaw. J Evid Based Dent Pract. 2012;**12**(3 Suppl):233-47.

[22] Landesberg R, Woo V, Cremers S, Cozin M, Marolt D, Vunjak-Novakovic G, et al. Potential pathophysiological mechanisms in osteonecrosis of the jaw. Ann N Y Acad Sci. 2011;**1218**(1):62-79.

[23] Reid IR, Bolland MJ, Grey AB. Is bisphosphonate-associated osteonecrosis of the jaw caused by soft tissue toxicity? Bone. 2007;**41**(3):318-20.

[24] Ohbayashi Y, Miyake M, Sawai F, Minami Y, Iwasaki A, Matsui Y. Adjunct teriparatide therapy with monitoring of bone turnover markers and bone scintigraphy for bisphosphonate-related osteonecrosis of the jaw. Oral Surg Oral Med Oral Pathol Oral Radiol. 2013;**115**(4):e31-7.

[25] Kakehashi H, Ando T, Minamizato T, Nakatani Y, Kawasaki T, Ikeda H, et al. Administration of teriparatide improves the symptoms of advanced bisphosphonate-related osteonecrosis of the jaw: preliminary findings. Int J Oral Maxillofac Surg. 2015;**44**(12):1558-64.

[26] Matsuo A, Hamada H, Takahashi H, Okamoto A, Kaise H, Chikazu D. Evaluation of dental implants as a risk factor for the development of bisphosphonate-related osteonecrosis of the jaw in breast cancer patients. Odontology. 2016;**104**(3):363-71.

[27] Holzinger D, Seemann R, Matoni N, Ewers R, Millesi W, Wutzl A. Effect of dental implants on bisphosphonate-related osteonecrosis of the jaws. J Oral Maxillofac Surg. 2014;**72**(10):1937.e1-8.

[28] Ramírez L, López-Pintor RM, Casañas E, Arriba L de, Hernández G. New non-bisphosphonate drugs that produce osteonecrosis of the jaws. Oral Health Prev Dent. 2015;**13**(5):385-93.

[29] Montefusco V, Gay F, Spina F, Miceli R, Maniezzo M, Teresa Ambrosini M, et al. Antibiotic prophylaxis before dental procedures may reduce the incidence of osteonecrosis of the jaw in patients with multiple myeloma treated with bisphosphonates. Leuk Lymphoma. 2008;**49**(11):2156-62.

[30] Kunchur R, Goss A. The oral health status of patients on oral bisphosphonates for osteoporosis. Aust Dent J. 2008;**53**(4):354-7.

[31] Ferlito S, Puzzo S, Liardo C. Preventive protocol for tooth extractions in patients treated with zoledronate: a case series. J Oral Maxillofac Surg. 2011;**69**(6):e1-4.

[32] Khan AA, Morrison A, Kendler DL, Rizzoli R, Hanley DA, Felsenberg D, et al. Case-based review of osteonecrosis of the jaw (ONJ) and application of the international recommendations for management from the international task force on ONJ. J Clin Densitom. 2016;**20**(1):8-24(Article in press).

[33] Allen MR. Medication-related osteonecrosis of the jaw. Oral Maxillofac Surg Clin North Am. 2015;**27**(4):497-508.

[34] Yamagata K, Nagai H, Baba O, Uchida F, Kanno N, Hasegawa S, et al. A Case of brain abscess caused by medication-related osteonecrosis of the jaw. Case Rep Dent. 2016;**2016**:1-4.